Fifth Edition

Study Guide for

Nursing

RESEARCH

Principles and Methods

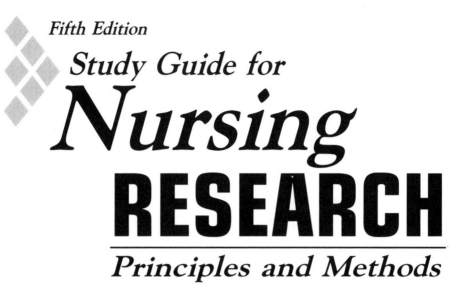

Fifth Edition

Study Guide for
Nursing
RESEARCH

Principles and Methods

Denise F. Polit, PH.D.
President
Humanalysis, Inc.
Saratoga Springs, New York

Bernadette P. Hungler, R.N., PH.D.
Associate Professor
Boston College School of Nursing
Chestnut Hill, Massachusetts

J. B. LIPPINCOTT COMPANY
Philadelphia

Sponsoring Editor: Margaret Belcher
Coordinating Editorial Assistant: Renee Gagliardi
Project Editor: Amy P. Jirsa
Design Coordinator: Doug Smock
Production Manager: Helen Ewan
Production Coordinator: Robert Randall
Compositor: The Composing Room of Michigan, Inc.
Printer/Binder: R. R. Donnelley & Sons Company
Cover Printer: Lehigh Presss

5th Edition

6 5 4 3 2

ISBN 0-397-55139-8

Any procedure or practice described in this book should be applied by the health-care practitioner under appropriate supervision in accordance with professional standards of care used with regard to the unique circumstances that apply in each practice situation. Care has been taken to confirm the accuracy of information presented and to describe generally accepted practices. However, the authors, editors, and publisher cannot accept any responsibility for errors or omissions or for any consequences from application of the information in this book and make no warranty express or implied, with respect to the contents of the book.

Every effort has been made to ensure drug selections and dosages are in accordance with current recommendations and practice. Because of ongoing research, changes in government regulations and the constant flow of information on drug therapy, reactions and interactions, the reader is cautioned to check the package insert for each drug for indications, dosages, warnings and precautions, particularly if the drug is new or infrequently used.

∞ Text printed on acid-free paper.

Preface

This Study Guide has been prepared to complement the fifth edition of *Nursing Research: Principles and Methods.* The guide provides opportunities to reinforce the acquisition of basic research skills through systematic learning exercises. The book is also intended to help bridge the gap between the passive reading of complex, abstract materials and active participation in the development of research skills through concrete examples and study suggestions.

As in the case of the textbook, this Study Guide was developed on the premise that research examples are a critical component of the learning process. The inclusion of actual and fictitious research examples is designed to instruct (i.e., facilitate the absorption of research concepts); motivate (i.e., encourage curiosity and an interest in acquiring research skills); and stimulate (i.e., suggest topics that might be pursued further by nurse researchers and practicing nurses interested in the utilization of research findings).

The Study Guide consists of 27 chapters—one chapter corresponding to every chapter in the textbook. Each of the 27 chapters consists of five sections:

- *Matching Exercises.* Terms and concepts presented in the textbook are reinforced by having students perform a matching routine that often involves matching the concrete (e.g., actual hypotheses) with the abstract (e.g., type of hypotheses).
- *Completion Exercises.* Sentences are presented in which the student must fill in a missing word or phrase corresponding to important ideas presented in the textbook.
- *Study Questions.* Each chapter contains several short individual exercises relevant to the materials in the textbook, including the preparation of definitions of terms.
- *Application Exercises.* These exercises, geared primarily to the consumers of nursing research, involve opportunities to critique various aspects of a study. Each chapter contains both fictitious research examples and suggestions for one or more actual research examples, which students are asked to evaluate according to a dimension emphasized in the corresponding chapter of the

textbook. A new feature of this edition is the inclusion of two complete studies for students' critical appraisal.

- *Special Projects.* This section, geared primarily to the producers of nursing research, offers suggestions for fairly large projects in which, in many cases, an entire classroom could collaborate.

Like the textbook, this Study Guide is expected to find application at both the undergraduate and graduate levels, and may be of heuristic value to practicing nurses as well.

Contents

Part V: The Analysis of Research Data

Part VI: Communication in the Research Process

Part VII: Research Reports

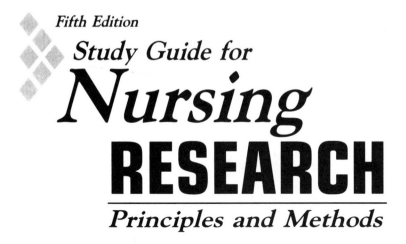

Fifth Edition

Study Guide for

Nursing

RESEARCH

Principles and Methods

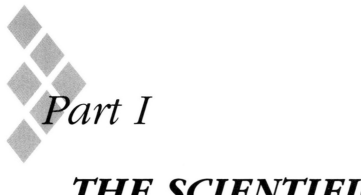

Part I

THE SCIENTIFIC RESEARCH PROCESS

Chapter 1

NURSING RESEARCH AND
THE SCIENTIFIC APPROACH

A. Matching Exercises

1. Match each of the activities in Set B with one of the timeframes in Set A. Indicate the letter corresponding to the appropriate response next to each entry in Set B.

SET A

a. Pre-1950s
b. 1950s
c. 1960s
d. 1970s
e. 1980s to present

SET B   **RESPONSE**

1. Nursing research focused on nurses themselves   _____
2. Increased research focus on clinical problems   _____
3. Establishment of the National Institute of Nursing Research at
   the National Institutes of Health   _____
4. Creation of the professional journal *Research in Nursing and
   Health*   _____
5. First nursing research study conducted   _____
6. Creation of the professional journal *Nursing Research*   _____
7. Increased interest in theoretical bases for conducting nursing
   research   _____
8. Establishment of a nursing archive at Boston University   _____
9. Nursing unit focusing on research established at Walter Reed   _____

10. Release of the Goldmark Report focusing on nursing educa-
    tion   _____

2. Match each of the research questions in Set B with one of the purposes for
conducting research in Set A. Indicate the letter corresponding to the appropriate
response next to each entry in Set B.

SET A
a. Description
b. Exploration
c. Explanation
d. Prediction/control

SET B   **RESPONSE**
1. What is the nature of the emotional experience of loneliness
   among the institutionalized elderly?   _____
2. What factors predict the use of contraceptives at first intercourse among teenaged women?   _____
3. What percentage of women fail to receive prenatal care during the first trimester of a pregnancy?   _____
4. What are the underlying causes of burnout among RNs working in intensive care units?   _____
5. What is the process by which terminally ill patients take leave
   of their families and close friends?   _____
6. What types of characteristics are related to a woman's decision to return to work within 6 weeks postpartum?   _____
7. Does vestibular stimulation affect the duration of quiet sleep
   among preterm infants?   _____
8. Why are teenaged mothers less likely to breastfeed their infants than older mothers?   _____

B. Completion Exercises

Write the words or phrases that correctly complete the sentences below.

1. Research in nursing began with _____

   _____ .

2. During the early years, most nursing studies focused on _____

   _____ .

3. The _____

   _____ , created by the American Nurses' Association, was founded for the promotion of nursing research.

4. The future direction of nursing research is likely to involve a continuing focus on

   _____

   _____ .

5. The approach to human knowledge that uses systematic, controlled procedures is known as the _____

   _____ .

6. The most ingrained source of knowledge, and the one that is the most difficult to challenge, is _____

   _____ .

7. The process of developing generalizations from specific observations is referred to as _____

   _____ reasoning.

8. Evidence that is rooted in objective reality and gathered through the human senses is known as _____

   _____ evidence.

9. The scientific assumption that all phenomena have antecedent causes is called

   _____

   _____ .

10. The characteristic of the scientific approach that enables researchers to rule out competing explanations is _____

    _____ .

11. Because scientific inquiry is not concerned with isolated phenomena, a key characteristic of the scientific method is _____

    _____ .

12. Of the various purposes of scientific inquiry, the one that epitomizes its spirit is

    _____

    _____ .

13. The type of research that involves the systematic collection and analysis of controlled, numerical information is known as _____

_____ .

14. The type of research that involves the systematic collection and analysis of subjective, narrative materials is known as _____

_____ .

15. The scientific approach has as its philosophical underpinnings a school of thought known as _____

_____ .

16. The philosophical perspective that has challenged the traditional scientific approach on the grounds that it is overly reductionist is known as the _____

_____

perspective.

C. Study Questions

1. Define the following terms. Compare your definition with the definition in Chapter 1 or in the glossary.

    a. Producer of nursing research: _____

    _____

    _____

    b. Consumer of nursing research: _____

    _____

    _____

    c. National Institute of Nursing Research: _____

    _____

    _____

    d. Scientific methods: _____

    _____

    _____

e. Empiricism: _____

_____

_____

f. Deductive reasoning: _____

_____

_____

g. Inductive reasoning: _____

_____

_____

h. Applied research: _____

_____

_____

i. Basic research: _____

_____

_____

j. Assumption: _____

_____

_____

k. Phenomenology: _____

_____

_____

2. Why is it important for nurses who will never conduct their own research to understand scientific methods?

3. What are some potential consequences to the profession of nursing if nurses stopped conducting their own research?

4. Many students have concerns about courses on research methods. Complete the following sentences, expressing as honestly as possible your own feelings about research, and discuss your concerns with your class.

a. I (am/am not) looking forward to this class on nursing research because: _

_____

_____

   b. I think that I would like a course in nursing research methods better if: ___

   _____

   _____

   c. I think that a class in nursing research (will/will not) improve my effective-
      ness as a nurse because: _____

   _____

   _____

5. Below are several research problems. For each, indicate whether you think it is
   primarily an applied or basic research question. Justify your response.

   a. Does movement tempo affect perception of the passage of time? _____

   _____

   _____

   b. Does follow-up by nurses improve patients' compliance with their medica-
      tion regimen? _____

   _____

   _____

   c. Does the ingestion of cranberry juice reduce urinary tract infections? _____

   _____

   _____

   d. Is sweat gland activity related to ACTH levels? _____

   _____

   _____

   e. Is pain perception associated with a person's locus of control (an aspect of
      personality)? _____

   _____

   _____

   f. Does the type of nursing curriculum affect attrition rates in schools of nursing?

   _____

   _____

   _____

g. Does nicotine affect postural muscle tremor? _____

_____

_____

h. Does the nurse/patient ratio affect nurses' job satisfaction? _____

_____

_____

6. Below are descriptions of several research problems. Indicate whether you think the problem is best suited to a qualitative or quantitative approach, and indicate why you think this is so.

   a. What is the decision-making process of AIDS patients seeking treatment?

   b. What effect does room temperature have on the colonization rate of bacteria in urinary catheters?

   c. What are the sources of stress among nursing home residents?

   d. Does therapeutic touch affect the vital signs of hospitalized patients?

   e. What is the process by which nursing students acquire a professional nursing identity?

   f. What are the effects of prenatal instruction on the labor and delivery outcomes of pregnant women?

   g. What are the health care needs of the homeless, and what are the barriers they face in having those needs met?

7. What are some of the limitations of quantitative research? What are some of the limitations of qualitative research? Which approach seems best suited to address problems in which you might be interested? Why is that?

D. Application Exercises

1. Singleton (1994)* studied the effect of the wording of communications on encouraging the elderly to come forward for a flu vaccination. All members of a

_____

*The example is fictitious.

senior citizens' center in a middle-sized community (a total of 500 elderly men and women) were sent a letter advising them that a flu epidemic was anticipated that season and that the elderly were especially likely to benefit from an immunization. Half of the members were sent a letter stressing the benefits of getting a flu shot. The other half of the members were sent a letter stressing the potential dangers of *not* getting a flu shot. To avoid any biases, a lottery-type system was used to determine who got which letter. All the elderly were advised that free immunizations would be available at a community health clinic over a 1-week period and that free transportation would also be made available to them. Singleton monitored the rates of coming forward for a flu shot among the two groups of elderly to assess whether one approach of encouragement was more persuasive than the other.

Consider the aspects of this study in relationship to the issues discussed in this chapter. To assist you in your review, here are some guiding questions:

a. Discuss the relevance of this study to nursing.
b. Do the features of this study correspond to the characteristics of the scientific approach? To what extent are the characteristics of order, control, empiricism, generalization, and theory represented in this example?
c. How would you characterize the purpose of this study? Is its major aim description, exploration, explanation, prediction, or control? Is there more than one purpose? Would you say this study is an example of basic or applied research?
d. Review the various limitations of the scientific method discussed in Chapter 1 and consider whether and how each applies to the study under consideration.
e. In this study, would it be more appropriate to collect and analyze qualitative or quantitative information? Why do you think this is so?

2. Below are several suggested research articles. Skim one or more of these articles and respond to questions a through e from Question D.1 in terms of an actual research study:

- Hartweg, D. L. (1993). Self-care actions of healthy middle-aged women to promote well-being. *Nursing Research, 42,* 221–227.
- Locsin, R. C. (1993). Time experience of selected institutionalized adult clients. *Clinical Nursing Research, 2,* 451–463.
- Tappen, R. M. (1994). The effect of skill training on functional abilities of nursing home residents with dementia. *Research in Nursing and Health, 17,* 159–166.
- Ziemer, M. M., & Pigeon, J. G. (1993). Skin changes and pain in the nipple during the first week of lactation. *Journal of Obstetric, Gynecologic, and Neonatal Nursing, 22,* 247–256.

E. Special Projects

1. Consider the following research statement:

   The purpose of this study is to understand why nurses are or are not satisfied with their jobs.

   The basic purpose of this study as stated is descriptive. Alter the statement in such a way as to design a study whose essential purpose is exploration; explanation; prediction; and control.

2. Think of the last "fact" you learned with respect to clinical nursing practice. Try to discover the ultimate source of this information. Was it tradition ("This is the way it's always been done")? Authority ("Dr. So-and-so said so")? Logical reasoning ("This has been inferred from previous observations")? Or scientific method ("An empirical investigation discovered this to be the case")?

Chapter 2

OVERVIEW OF THE
RESEARCH PROCESS

A. MATCHING EXERCISES

1. Match each of the terms in Set B with one (or more) of the terms in Set A. Indicate the letter corresponding to your response next to each item in Set B.

SET A
a. Categorical variable
b. Continuous variable
c. Active variable
d. Attribute variable
e. Constant

SET B   **RESPONSE**

  1. Employment status (working/not working)   _____

  2. Dosage of a new drug   _____

  3. Pi (π—to calculate area of a circle)   _____

  4. Number of times hospitalized   _____

  5. Method of teaching patients (structured versus unstructured)   _____

  6. Blood type   _____

  7. pH level of urine   _____

  8. Pulse rate of a deceased person   _____

  9. Membership in a nursing union   _____

10. Birthweight of an infant   _____

Polit DF, Hungler BP: STUDY GUIDE FOR NURSING RESEARCH:
PRINCIPLES AND METHODS, 5th ed. © 1995 J.B. Lippincott Company.

11. Presence or absence of decubitus   _____
12. Degree of empathy in nurses   _____

2. Match each of the terms in Set B with one of the terms in Set A. Indicate the letter corresponding to your response next to each item in Set B.

SET A
a. Independent variable
b. Dependent variable
c. Either/both

SET B   **RESPONSE**
 1. The variable that is the presumed effect   _____
 2. The variable that is dichotomous   _____
 3. The variable that is the main outcome of interest in the study _____
 4. The variable that is the presumed cause   _____
 5. The variable referred to as the criterion variable   _____
 6. The variable that is an attribute   _____
 7. The variable, "length of stay in hospital"   _____
 8. The variable that requires an operational definition   _____

B. Completion Exercises

Write the words or phrases that correctly complete the sentences below.

 1. The person who is the leader of a team of researchers is known as the _____
    _____ or _____ .

 2. The people who are being studied in a research project are referred to as the
    _____ or _____
    _____ .

 3. The abstract qualities in which a researcher is interested are referred to in scientific parlance as _____ or _____
    _____ .

 4. The variable that the researcher wants to understand, explain, or predict is
    known as the _____ or _____
    _____ variable.

5. The variable presumed to *cause* or influence changes in some other variable is the _____ .

6. If a researcher studied the effect of a scheduling assignment on nurses' morale, scheduling assignment would be referred to as the _____ _____ variable.

7. Whereas gender is a categorical variable, height is a(n) _____ _____ variable.

8. When a researcher carefully specifies the steps that must be taken to measure the concepts of interest, she or he develops _____ _____ .

9. The pieces of information obtained in the course of a study are collectively known as the _____ _____ .

10. "The higher the caloric intake, the greater the weight" expresses a presumed ____ _____

relationship.

11. "Men are more likely to be noncompliant with a medication regimen than women" expresses a presumed _____ _____ relationship.

12. A variable that is irrelevant in an investigation and needs to be controlled is called a(n) _____ _____ variable.

13. The researcher's expectations about how variables under investigation are related are stated in the _____ _____ .

14. The overall plan for structuring a study is called the _____ _____ .

15. Research in which the investigator plays an active, interventive role is called

_____

_____ research.

16. The total aggregate of units that a researcher is interested in is known as the

_____

_____ .

17. The two basic categories of sampling are referred to as _____

_____ and _____ sampling.

18. The actual group of study participants selected from a larger group is known as

the _____

_____ .

19. The primary criterion by which a sample is assessed for adequacy is its _____

_____ of the

population.

20. Typically, the most time-consuming phase of the study is the _____

_____ phase.

21. A small-scale trial run of a research study is referred to as a(n) _____

_____ .

22. The plan for transforming research information into a numerical format suitable

for analysis is called the _____

_____ .

23. The task of organizing the information collected in a study is known as _____

_____ .

24. The two broad classes of analysis are referred to as _____

and _____ analysis.

25. The final phase of a research project is known as the _____

_____ phase.

C. Study Questions

1. Define the following concepts. Compare your definition with the definition in Chapter 2 or in the glossary.

   a. Investigator: _____

   _____

   _____

   b. Subject: _____

   _____

   _____

   c. Construct: _____

   _____

   _____

   d. Variable: _____

   _____

   _____

   e. Heterogeneity: _____

   _____

   _____

   f. Categorical variable: _____

   _____

   _____

   g. Operational definition: _____

   _____

   _____

   h. Relationship: _____

   _____

   _____

i. Cause-and-effect relationship: _____

_____

_____

j. Functional relationship: _____

_____

_____

k. Research control: _____

_____

_____

l. Mediating variable: _____

_____

_____

m. Data collection plan: _____

_____

_____

n. Sampling plan: _____

_____

_____

2. Suggest operational definitions for the following concepts.

a. Stress: _____

_____

_____

b. Prematurity of infants: _____

_____

_____

c. Nursing effectiveness: _____

_____

_____

d. Knowledge of critical care nursing concepts: _____

_____

_____

e. Nurses' educational preparation: _____

_____

_____

f. Patient recovery: _____

_____

_____

g. Prolonged labor: _____

_____

_____

h. Smoking behavior: _____

_____

_____

i. Nurses' job dissatisfaction: _____

_____

_____

j. Respiratory function: _____

_____

_____

3. In each of the following research problems, identify the independent and dependent variables.

a. Does assertiveness training improve the effectiveness of psychiatric nurses?

Independent: _____

Dependent: _____

b. Does the postural positioning of patients affect their respiratory function?

Independent: _____

Dependent: _____

c. Is the psychological well-being of patients affected by the amount of touch received from nursing staff?

Independent: _____

Dependent: _____

d. Is the incidence of decubitus reduced by more frequent turnings of patients?

Independent: _____

Dependent: _____

e. Is the educational preparation of nurses related to their subsequent turnover rate?

Independent: _____

Dependent: _____

f. Is tolerance for pain related to a patient's age and gender?

Independent: _____

Dependent: _____

g. Are the number of prenatal visits of pregnant women associated with labor and delivery outcomes?

Independent: _____

Dependent: _____

h. Are levels of stress among nurses higher in pediatric or adult intensive care units?

Independent: _____

Dependent: _____

i. Are student nurses' clinical grades related to their subsequent on-the-job performances?

Independent: _____

Dependent: _____

j. Is anxiety in surgical patients affected by structured preoperative teaching?

Independent: _____

Dependent: _____

k. Are nurses' promotions related to their level of participation in continuing education activities?

    Independent: _____

    Dependent: _____

l. Does hearing acuity of the elderly change as a function of the time of day?

    Independent: _____

    Dependent: _____

m. Is patient satisfaction with nursing care related to the congruity of nurses' and patients' cultural backgrounds?

    Independent: _____

    Dependent: _____

n. Is a woman's educational background related to breast self-examination practices?

    Independent: _____

    Dependent: _____

o. Does home birth affect the parents' satisfaction with the childbirth experience?

    Independent: _____

    Dependent: _____

4. For each of the variables in Question C.3, indicate which is a categorical variable and which is a continuous variable.

5. Below is a list of variables. For each, think of a research problem for which the variable would be the independent variable, and a second for which it would be the dependent variable. For example, take the variable "birthweight of infants." We might ask, "Does the age of the mother affect the birthweight of her infant?" (dependent variable). Alternatively, we could define our research question as, "Does the birthweight of infants (independent variable) affect their sensorimotor development at 6 months of age?" HINT: For the dependent variable problem, ask yourself, What factors might affect, influence, or cause this variable? For the independent variable, ask yourself, What factors does *this* variable influence, cause, or affect?

a. Body temperature

    Independent: _____

    Dependent: _____

b. Amount of sleep

Independent: _____

Dependent: _____

c. Frequency of practicing breast self examination

Independent: _____

Dependent: _____

d. Level of hopefulness in cancer patients

Independent: _____

Dependent: _____

e. Amount of saliva secretion

Independent: _____

Dependent: _____

f. Nurses' absentee rate

Independent: _____

Dependent: _____

D. Application Exercises

1. Nicolet (1995)* observed that different patients react differently to sensory over-load in the hospital. She conducted a study to see whether the patients' home environments affect their reactions to hospital noises. Below are the investigator's operational definitions of the research variables.

   Independent Variable: Type of home environment: Based on the patients' self-reports at intake, home environment was defined as the number of house-hold members residing with the patient.

   Dependent Variable: Reaction to hospital noise: Based on responses to five questions (agree/disagree type) answered at discharge, patients were clas-sified as "dissatisfied with noise level" or "not dissatisfied with noise level."

   Extraneous Variables

   Age: calculated to the nearest year based on information on date of birth reported at intake

   Gender: patient's gender as recorded on intake form

   Social class: patient's occupation as recorded on intake form

*This example is fictitious.

Review and comment on these specifications. Suggest alternatives, and compare the adequacy and completeness of your suggestions with the descriptions provided above. To aid you in this task, here are some guiding questions:

   a. Are the operational definitions sufficiently detailed? Do they tell the reader exactly how each variable is to be measured? Can you expand any of the definitions so that they are more precise?

   b. Are the operational definitions good definitions—that is, is there a better way to measure, say, home environment?

   c. Has the researcher identified reasonable extraneous variables—that is, are these extraneous variables likely to be related to both the dependent and independent variables?

   d. Are there extraneous variables that the researcher failed to identify but that should be controlled? Suggest two or three additional extraneous variables.

2. Below are several suggested research articles. Read one of these articles and identify the independent variable(s) and dependent variable(s) of the study. Also, respond to questions a through d from Question D.1 with regard to this actual research study.

   • Beach, E. K., Maloney, B. H., Plocica, A. R., Sherry, S. E., Weaver, M., Luthringer, L., & Utz, S. (1992). The spouse: A factor in recovery after acute myocardial infarction. *Heart and Lung, 21,* 30–38.

   • Fuller, B. F., Keefe, M. R., & Curtin, B. J. (1994). Acoustic analysis of cries from "normal" and "irritable" infants. *Western Journal of Nursing Research, 16,* 243–250.

   • Mock, V. (1993). Body image in women treated for breast cancer. *Nursing Research, 42,* 153–157.

   • DiIorio, C., Faherty, B., & Manteuffel, B. (1992). Self-efficacy and social support in self-management of epilepsy. *Western Journal of Nursing Research, 14,* 292–303.

E. Special Projects

1. Suppose you were interested in studying the effect of a hysterectomy on women's sexuality and sexual identity. Briefly outline what you might do in the following tasks, as outlined in this chapter:

   Step 4   Formulate hypotheses: _____

   _____

   _____

   Step 5   Select a research design: _____

   _____

   _____

Step 6   Identify the population: _____

_____

_____

Step 7   Specify the methods to measure or operationalize the variables: _____

_____

_____

Step 8   Select a sample: _____

_____

_____

2. Now suppose that, for the study you have described above, you needed to prepare a schedule for the completion of Steps 2 through 15. Assume you have 12 months to complete the study. Prepare a time schedule for the 14 tasks on the chart below:

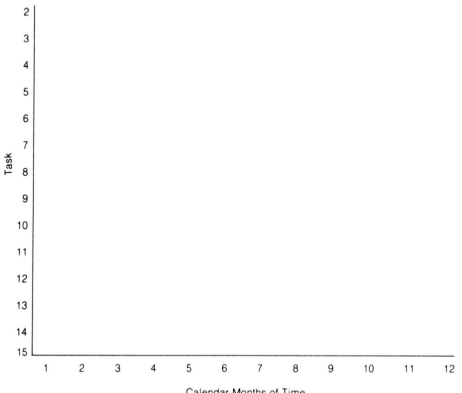

3. Another researcher is investigating the effect of auditory versus tactile stimulation on the crying behavior of premature infants. Ten babies are exposed to soft music for 5 minutes, four times a day. Ten other babies are exposed to extra touching and caressing for 5 minutes, four times a day. The dependent variable is the total number of minutes of crying among these infants for the 5 days of the treatment. Indicate a time schedule for this project, superimposed on the chart above, in a different color ink or pencil. Compare the differences between the two projects in time spent on various tasks. Justify the differences.

Chapter 3

RESEARCH PROBLEMS
AND HYPOTHESES

A. MATCHING EXERCISES

Match each of the statements in Set B with one of the terms in Set A. Indicate the letter corresponding to the appropriate response next to each statement in Set B.

SET A
a. Research hypothesis–directional
b. Research hypothesis—nondirectional
c. Null hypothesis
d. Not a hypothesis as stated

SET B	RESPONSE
1. First-born infants have higher concentrations of estrogens and progesterone in umbilical cord blood than do later-born infants.	_____
2. There is no relationship between participation in prenatal classes and the health outcomes of infants.	_____
3. Nursing students are increasingly interested in obtaining advanced degrees.	_____
4. Nurse practitioners have more job mobility than do other registered nurses.	_____
5. A person's age is related to his or her difficulty in accessing health care.	_____

6. Glaucoma can be effectively screened by means of tonome-
   try.   _____

7. Increased noise levels result in increased anxiety among hospitalized patients.   _____

8. Media exposure of the health hazards of smoking is unrelated
   to the public's smoking habits.   _____

9. Nurses' job satisfaction is correlated with levels of occupational stress.   _____

10. The primary reason that nurses participate in continuing edu-
    cation programs is for professional advancement.   _____

11. Baccalaureate, diploma, and associate degree nursing gradu-
    ates differ with respect to technical and clinical skills ac-
    quired.   _____

12. Nurses' experiences with abortion patients have no effect on
    the nurses' attitudes toward abortion.   _____

13. Nurses' shift assignments are associated with their rates of
    absenteeism.   _____

14. The presence of homonymous hemianopia in stroke patients
    negatively affects their length of stay in hospital.   _____

15. Adjustment to hemodialysis does not vary by the patient's
    sex.   _____

B. Completion Exercises

Write the words or phrases that correctly complete the sentences below.

1. The four most common sources of ideas for research problems are

   _____ , _____ , _____ , _____ , and

   _____ .

2. Unavailability of subjects would make a research project _____

   _____ .

3. Moral or philosophical questions are inherently _____

   _____ .

4. Adequacy of research facilities and time bear on the _____

   _____ of the research project.

5. In order to be researchable, the variables in a research project need to be _____

_____ .

6. The form of the problem statement can be either _____

_____ or _____ .

7. Research hypotheses state a predicted _____

_____ between variables.

8. Hypotheses normally should be formulated _____

_____ data collection.

9. A hypothesis involves a prediction regarding at least _____

_____ variables.

10. Another term for complex hypothesis is _____

_____ .

11. The _____

_____ hypothesis states that there is no expected relationship among the
research variables.

12. Hypotheses are generally tested by means of _____

_____ .

13. Hypotheses predict the effect of the _____
variable on the _____ variable.

14. Theories form the basis for _____ hypotheses through the process of _____ .

C. Study Questions

1. Define the following terms. Compare your definition with the definition in Chapter 3 of the textbook or in the glossary.

a. Problem statement: _____

_____

_____

b. Statement of purpose: _____

_____

_____

c. Research question: _____

_____

_____

d. Unresearchable problem: _____

_____

_____

e. Unfeasible problem: _____

_____

_____

f. Hypothesis: _____

_____

_____

g. Inductive hypothesis: _____

_____

_____

h. Deductive hypothesis: _____

_____

_____

i. Simple hypothesis: _____

_____

_____

j. Complex hypothesis: _____

_____

_____

k. Nondirectional hypothesis: _____

_____

_____

l. Null Hypothesis: _____

_____

_____

m. Directional hypothesis: _____

_____

_____

2. Each of the problem statements below is either unresearchable or unfeasible as stated. Reword the statements, maintaining the general theme, such that a researchable and feasible problem is developed.

ORIGINAL

REWORDED

a. What is the best approach for dealing with family members of a dying patient?

b. Should surrogate motherhood be forbidden by law?

c. Should retirement for nurses be mandatory at age 65?

d. Should abortion be available on demand?

e. How can nurses be encouraged to do their own research?

f. What is the best procedure for reducing stress among children before immunization?

g. What incentives will motivate nursing faculty to publish professional articles?

h. What role can humor play in improving the well-being of the institutionalized elderly?

3. Below is a list of general topics that could be investigated. Develop at least one problem statement for each. Assess the adequacy of your statement in terms of the problem's researchability and the wording of the statement. HINT: Think of these concepts as potential independent or dependent variables. Ask: What might cause or affect this variable? and, What might be the consequences or effects of this variable? This should lead to some ideas for a problem statement. Also, review the question items in the section in the textbook called Narrowing the Topic.

a. Patient comfort: _____

_____

_____

b. Psychiatric patients' readmission rates: _____

_____

_____

c. Anxiety in hospitalized children: _____

_____

_____

d. Elevated blood pressure: _____

_____

_____

e. Nurses' job satisfaction: _____

_____

_____

f. Patient cooperativeness in the recovery room: _____

_____

_____

g. Nutritional knowledge: _____

_____

_____

h. Mother–infant bonding: _____

_____

_____

i. Menstrual irregularities: _____

_____

_____

4. Below is a list of researchable problem statements. Transform those stated in the interrogative form to the declarative form, and vice versa.

ORIGINAL VERSION

TRANSFORMED VERSION

a. Can a program of nursing counseling affect sexual readjustment among women after a hysterectomy?

_____

b. The purpose of the research is to study the relationship between nurses' unit assignments and their absentee rates.

_____

c. What are the sequelae of an inadequately maintained sterile environment for tracheal suctioning?

_____

d. What is the relationship between Type A/Type B personalities and speech patterns?

_____

e. The purpose of the study is to examine the effect of an AIDS education workshop on teenagers' understanding of AIDS and the HIV virus.

_____

f. The purpose of the research is to study patients' response to transfer from a coronary care unit to a general care unit.

_____

g. What effect does the presence of the father in the delivery room have on the mother's satisfaction with the childbirth experience?

_____

h. The purpose of the study is to examine the effect of clients' physical proximity to community health centers on health care utilization.

_____

i. What is the long-term child development effect of maternal heroin addiction during pregnancy?

_____

j. The purpose of the research is to study the effect of spermicides on the physiologic development of the fetus.

_____

5. Below are five nondirectional hypotheses. Restate each one as a directional hypothesis.

NONDIRECTIONAL

a. Nurses' attitudes toward mental retardation vary according to their clinical specialty area.

b. Nurses and patients differ in terms of the relative importance they attach to having the patients' physical versus emotional needs met.

c. Type of nursing care (primary versus team) is unrelated to patient satisfaction with the care received.

d. The incidence of decubitus ulcers is related to the frequency of turning patients.

e. Baccalaureate and associate degree nurses differ in use of touch as a therapeutic device with patients.

DIRECTIONAL

_____

_____

_____

_____

_____

6. Below are five simple hypotheses. Change each one to a complex hypothesis by adding either a dependent or independent variable.

SIMPLE HYPOTHESIS

a. First-time blood donors experience greater stress during the donation than donors who have given blood previously.

b. Nurses who initiate more conversation with patients are rated as more effective in their nursing care by patients than those who initiate less conversation.

c. Surgical patients who give high ratings to the informativeness of nursing communications experience less preoperative stress than do patients who give low ratings.

d. Appendectomy patients whose peritoneums are drained with a Penrose drain will experience

COMPLEX HYPOTHESIS

_____

_____

_____

more peritoneal infection than patients who are not drained.

_____

e. Women who give birth by cesarean section are more likely to experience postpartum depression than women who give birth vaginally.

_____

7. In study questions 5 and 6 above, 10 research hypotheses were provided. Identify the independent and dependent variables in each.

INDEPENDENT VARIABLE(S)	DEPENDENT VARIABLE(S)
5a	
5b	
5c	
5d	
5e	
6a	
6b	
6c	
6d	
6e	

8. Below are five statements that are *not* research hypotheses as currently stated. Suggest modifications to these statements that would make them testable research hypotheses.

ORIGINAL STATEMENT   **HYPOTHESIS**

a. Relaxation therapy is effective in reducing hypertension.

_____

b. The use of bilingual health care staff produces high utilization rates of health care facilities by ethnic minorities.

_____

c. Nursing students are affected in their choice of clinical specialization by interactions with nursing faculty.

_____

d. Sexually active teenagers have a high rate of using male methods of contraception.

_____

e. In-use intravenous solutions become contaminated within 48 hours.

_____

9. Review the major purposes of a research hypothesis. In light of these purposes, explain why the null hypothesis is of less utility in the early phases of a scientific study than a research hypothesis.

D. *Application Exercises*

1. Matysik (1994)* was interested in studying the effects of a mutual help group for widows and widowers. She designed a study in which 25 people who had lost a spouse 6 to 12 months earlier participated in biweekly mutual help group sessions. A comparison group of 25 nonparticipating widows and widowers was also included in the study. Matysik was interested in evaluating the effect of participation on several indexes of socioemotional well-being. The aim of her investigation was to answer the following questions:

   • Does participation in a mutual help group improve the bereaved's morale?
   • Does participation in a mutual help group reduce feelings of social isolation?
   • Does participation in a mutual help group affect self-esteem?
   • Does participation in a mutual help group lead to better acceptance of the spouse's death?

   Review and critique these problem statements. Suggest alternatives and/or supplementary problem statements. To assist you, here are some guiding questions:

   a. How adequate are these problem statements in terms of researchability? Do they communicate the intent of the study? Can you alter the statements so that they are more precise or more amenable to research?

   b. Given the overall intent of the study, are the four specific research questions a good, well-balanced representation? (That is, are the four dependent variables good indicators of "socioemotional well-being"?) Can you develop additional research questions that would extend the overall goal of the project?

   c. What obstacles to the study's feasibility should the researcher consider?

2. Below are several suggested research articles. Read the introductory sections of one or more of these articles and respond to questions a through c from Question D.1 in terms of these actual research studies:

   • Belza, B. L., Henke, C. J., Yelin, E. H., Epstein, W. V., & Gilliss, C. L. (1993). Correlates of fatigue in older adults with rheumatoid arthritis. *Nursing Research, 42,* 93–99.
   • Brown, M. A., & Powell-Cope, G. (1993). Themes of loss and dying in caring for a family member with AIDS. *Research in Nursing and Health, 16,* 179–191.

*This example is fictitious.

- Dick, M. J. (1993). Preterm infants in pain: Nurses' and physicians perceptions. *Clinical Nursing Research, 2,* 176–187.
- Scott, C. B. (1992). Circular victimization in the caregiving relationship. *Western Journal of Nursing Research, 15,* 230–245.

3. Ribeiro (1995)† was interested in studying the notes made by various members of the health care team on patients' hospital charts. The investigator was concerned with several aspects of the chart in terms of its communication potential to various hospital personnel. She began her project with some general questions, such as: Are the nurses' entries on the patient chart used by other staff? Who is most likely to read nurses' entries on the chart? Are there particular types of medical conditions that encourage staff utilization of nurses' entries? Do particular types of entries encourage utilization?   Ribeiro proceeded to reflect on her own experiences and observations relative to these issues and reviewed the literature to find whether other researchers had addressed these problems. Based on her review and reflections, Ribeiro developed the following hypotheses:

- Nursing notes on patients' charts are referred to infrequently by hospital personnel.
- Physicians refer to nursing notes on the patients' charts less frequently than do other personnel.
- The use of nursing notes by physicians is related to the location of the notes on the chart.
- Nurses perceive that nursing notes are referred to less frequently than is the case.
- Nursing notes are more likely to be referred to by hospital personnel if the patient has been hospitalized for more than 5 days than if the patient has been hospitalized for 5 days or fewer.

Review and critique these hypotheses. Suggest alternative wordings or supplementary hypotheses. To assist you, here are some guiding questions:

   a. Are all the hypotheses testable as stated? What changes (if any) are needed to make all the hypotheses testable?

   b. Are the hypotheses all consistent in format and style? That is, are they directional, nondirectional, or stated in the null form? Suggest changes, if appropriate, that would make them consistent.

   c. Are the above hypotheses reasonable (i.e., logical and consistent with your own experience and observations)? Are the hypotheses significant (i.e., do they have the potential to contribute to the nursing profession)?

†This example is fictitious.

    d. Based on the general problem that the researcher identified, can you generate additional hypotheses that could be tested? Can you suggest modifications to the hypotheses above to make them complex rather than simple (i.e., introduce additional independent or dependent variables)?

4. Below are several suggested research articles. Read the introductory sections of one or more of these articles and respond to questions a through d from Question D.3 in terms of these actual research studies:

- Barkman, A., & Lunse, C. P. (1994). The effect of early ambulation on patient comfort and delayed bleeding after cardiac angiogram. *Heart and Lung, 23,* 112–117.

- Howell, R. D., MacRae, L. D., Sanjines, S., Burke, J., & DeStefano, P. (1992). Effects of two types of head coverings in the rewarming of patients after coronary artery bypass graft surgery. *Heart and Lung, 21,* 1–5.

- Maikler, V. E. (1991). Effects of a skin refrigerant/anesthetic and age on the pain responses of infants receiving immunizations. *Research in Nursing and Health, 14,* 397–402.

- Nyamathi, A., Jacoby, A., Constancia, P., & Ruvevich, S. (1992). Coping and adjustment of spouses of critically ill patients with cardiac disease. *Heart and Lung, 21,* 160–166.

- Van Riper, M., Ryff, C., & Pridham, K. (1992). Parental and family well-being in families of children with Down syndrome: A comparative study. *Research in Nursing and Health, 15,* 227–235.

E. Special Projects

1. Think of your clinical experience as a student or practicing nurse. Consider some aspect of your work that you particularly enjoy. Is there anything about that part of your work that puzzles, intrigues, or frustrates you? Can you conceive of any procedure, practice, or information that would improve the quality of your work in that area or improve the care you provide? Ask yourself a series of similar questions until a general problem area emerges. Narrow the problem area until you have a workable research problem statement. Assess the problem in terms of the criteria of significance, researchability, feasibility, and interest to you.

2. Read the article by Kuhlman and her colleagues (1991) entitled "Alzheimer's disease and family caregiving: Critical synthesis of the literature and research agenda," in *Nursing Research,* volume 40, issue 6 (or read some other research review article). Based on the author's summary of prior research, develop a problem statement for a study that would extend knowledge about Alzheimer's disease family caregiving. Assess your problem statement in terms of the criteria of significance, researchability, feasibility, and personal interest.

3. Below are two sets of variables. Select a variable from each set to generate directional hypotheses. In other words, use one variable in Set A as the independent variable and one variable in Set B as the dependent variable (or vice versa), and make a prediction about the relationship between the two.‡ Generate five hypotheses in this fashion.

SET A
Body temperature
Patients' level of hopefulness
Attitudes toward death
Frequency of medications
Delivery by nurse midwife versus physician
Participation in continuing education courses
Years of nursing experience
Amount of interaction between nurses and patients' families
Preoperative anxiety levels
Patients' amount of privacy during hospitalization
Smoking status (smokes versus does not smoke)
Recidivism in a psychiatric hospital

SET B
Patient satisfaction with nursing care
Nurses' educational preparation
Infant Apgar score
Attitudes toward nursing research
Effectiveness of nursing care
Nursing specialty area
Patients' compliance with nursing instructions
Nurses' part-time versus full-time work schedules
Nurses' ages
Nurses' empathy
Hospital staff morale
Patients' pulse rates

Assess the hypotheses generated in terms of significance, testability, and interest to you.

‡As one example: Pregnant women who smoke will give birth to babies with lower Apgar scores than women who do not smoke.

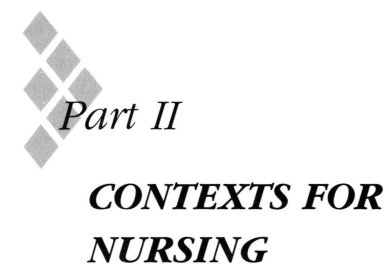

Part II

CONTEXTS FOR NURSING RESEARCH

Chapter 4

THE KNOWLEDGE CONTEXT: LITERATURE REVIEWS

A. MATCHING EXERCISES

Below, under Set B, are a number of fictitious references from the *International Nursing Index*. Identify the portion of the reference that is <u>underlined</u> and match it with a term in Set A. Indicate the letter corresponding to the appropriate response next to each entry in Set B.

SET A

a. Journal
b. Volume
c. Pages
d. Issue
e. Author
f. Title

SET B   **RESPONSE**

1. Convalescence following a hysterectomy. Sprunk, K. <u>Nurs Res</u> 1993 May–June; 42(2): 157–162.   _____

2. Nursing care program for bed-confined patients. <u>Colangelo, B.</u> Nurs Clin North Am 1993 Jan; 28(1): 83–96.   _____

3. Nurse counseling following an abortion. Mazula, G. J Adv Nurs 1992 Nov; 9(<u>6</u>): 350–357.   _____

4. Level of activation and respiratory function. Griese, R. Nurs Res 1991 July; 40(4): <u>196–202</u>.   _____

5. Holistic care in a community health center. Kuczek, J. Nurs Clin North Am 1993 Feb; 29(2): 101–115.   _____

6. Treating bacteriuria in female patients with indwelling cathe-ters. Dizney, D. Nurs Outlook 1991 Dec; 33(12):770–779.   _____

7. Coping styles among children with diabetes. Vito, G. Clin Nurs Res 1993 Jan; 2(1): 15–20.   _____

8. Screening for scoliosis in school-age children. Gregory, T. J. Sch Health 1992 Mar; 59(5): 315–319.   _____

B. Completion Exercises

Write the words or phrases that correctly complete the sentences below.

1. The two types of information that have the least utility in a research review are _____ and _____ _____ .

2. The most important type of information to be included in a written research review is _____ _____ .

3. No hypothesis or theory can be definitively _____ _____ or _____ by the scientific method.

4. For students who are just beginning to engage in their own research, the most important function of the literature review is likely to be as a source of _____ _____ .

5. The most relevant index for materials specific to nursing is the _____ _____ .

6. When a computer search yields many references, the references are generally produced _____ _____ .

7. The computer database most often used in literature searches by nurses is _____ _____ .

8. The type of research reports that students are most likely to read are _____

_____ .

9. The oldest scholarly journal that has served as an outlet for nurses engaged in

scientific research is _____

_____ .

10. The six sections typically found in research journal articles are: _____ ,

_____ , _____ , _____ , _____ , and

_____ .

11. Quantity of references is less important in a good literature review than the

_____

_____ of the references.

12. The written literature review should paraphrase materials and use a minimum of

_____

_____ .

13. The literature review should make clear not only what is known about a problem

but also any _____

_____ in the research.

14. The review should conclude with a _____

_____ .

15. The literature review should be written in a language of _____

_____ , in keeping with

the limitations of available methods.

C. Study Questions

1. Define the following terms. Compare your definition with the definition in Chapter 4 of the textbook or in the glossary.

   a. Literature review: _____

   _____

   _____

b. Primary source: _____

_____

_____

c. Secondary source: _____

_____

_____

d. Key word: _____

_____

_____

e. Index: _____

_____

_____

f. Abstract journal: _____

_____

_____

g. On-line search: _____

_____

_____

h. End-user system: _____

_____

_____

i. Journal article: _____

_____

_____

2. Below are fictitious excerpts from research literature reviews. Each excerpt has a stylistic problem. Change each sentence to make it acceptable stylistically.

ORIGINAL	**REVISED**
a. Most elderly people do not eat a balanced diet.	_____
b. Patient characteristics have a significant impact on nursing workload.	_____

c. A child's conception of appropriate sick role behavior changes as the child grows older.

d. Home birth poses many potential dangers.

e. Multiple sclerosis results in considerable anxiety to the family of the patients.

f. Studies have proved that most nurses prefer not to work the night shift.

g. Life changes are the major cause of stress in adults.

h. Stroke rehabilitation programs are most effective when they involve the patients' families.

i. It has been proved that psychiatric outpatients have higher than average rates of accidental deaths and suicides.

j. Nursing faculty are increasingly involved in conducting their own research.

k. The traditional pelvic examination is sufficiently unpleasant to many women that they avoid having the examination.

l. It is known that most tonsillectomies performed three decades ago were unnecessary.

m. Few smokers seriously try to break the smoking habit.

n. Severe cutaneous burns often result in hemorrhagic gastric erosions.

3. Below are several problem statements. Indicate one or more key words that you would use to begin a literature search on this topic.

PROBLEM STATEMENT   **KEY WORDS**

a. How effective are nurse practitioners compared with pediatricians with respect to telephone management of acute pediatric illness?

b. Does contingency contracting improve patient compliance with a treatment regimen?

_____

c. Does induced abortion affect the outcome of subsequent pregnancies?

_____

d. Is the amount of money a person spends on food related to the adequacy of nutrient intake?

_____

e. Is rehabilitation after spinal cord injury affected by the age and occupation of the patient?

_____

f. Does the leadership style of head nurses affect the job tension and job performance of the nursing staff?

_____

g. Is loss of appetite among cancer patients associated with reactions to chemotherapy?

_____

h. What is the effect of alcohol skin preparation before insulin injection on the incidence of local and systemic infection?

_____

i. Are bottle-fed babies introduced to solid foods sooner than breast-fed babies?

_____

j. Do children raised on vegetarian diets have different growth patterns than other children?

_____

D. Application Exercises

1. Below is an excerpt from Nudo's (1994)* literature review dealing with pelvic inflammatory disease.

There are no universally accepted criteria for defining pelvic inflammatory disease (PID) or for categorizing its severity. Furthermore, PID does not exhibit uniformity in its clinical features. Etiologically, cases of acute PID can be divided on the basis of those caused by *Neisseria gonorrhoeae,* those caused by nongonococcal bacteria, and those caused by a combination of both. Eschenbach and his colleagues (1980) reported that about half of the women with PID whom they examined had gonococcal infections. Eschenbach (1985) noted that "this difference in etiological agents may explain the clinical differences between the gonococcal and nongonococcal PID. The latter may

*This example is fictitious.

appear less acute and may not demonstrate many of the well-defined clinical features associated with gonorrhea" (p. 148). Both gonococcal and nongonococcal PID may result in subsequent obstruction of the fallopian tubes, which is among the most common causes of infertility in women. Because fertilized eggs remain in the fallopian tubes for about 3 days, they must provide nourishment for the developing zygote. Thus, even a tube that is not completely blocked, but which is severely damaged, can contribute to infertility.

Westrom (1989), in a study of women treated for PID, proved that PID has an impact on subsequent fertility. A sample of 415 women with laparoscopically confirmed PID were reviewed after 9.5 years and compared with 100 control subjects who had never been treated for PID. Among the 415 women who had had PID, 88 (21.2%) were involuntarily childless; of these 88, the failure to conceive was due to tubal obstruction in 72 cases (82%). A total of 263 of the 415 subjects (63.4%) had become pregnant. In the control group, only three women (3%) were involuntarily childless.

Westrom's study also revealed a relationship between infertility and the number of PID infections. Tubal occlusion was diagnosed after one infection in 32 women (12.8%); after two infections in 22 cases (35.5%); and after three or more infections in 18 cases (75.0%). Of the 415 women with acute PID in Westrom's sample, 94 (22.7%) experienced more than one infection. Evidence from other studies confirms that a large percentage of women with PID have a history of previous PID and that recurrent PID usually has a nongonococcal etiology (Jacobson & Westrom, 1984; Ringrose, 1980; Eschenbach, 1987).

The number of women affected by PID annually in the United States is unknown and difficult to estimate. According to Rose (1983), Eschenbach and colleagues used data from the National Disease and Therapeutic Index Study and the Hospital Record Study to estimate that over 500,000 cases of PID occurred annually in the United States in the early 1970s. The information from the Hospital Record Study indicated that a mean of over 160,000 patients with PID were hospitalized annually from 1970 through 1973.

Critique this literature review regarding the points made in Chapter 4 of the textbook. To assist you in this task, here are some guiding questions:

a. Is the review well organized? Does the author skip from theme to theme in a disjointed way, or is there a logic to the order of presentation of materials?

b. Is the content of the review appropriate? Did the author use secondary sources when a primary source was available? Are all the references relevant, or does the inclusion of some material appear contrived? Do you have a sense that the author was thorough in uncovering all the relevant materials? Do the references seem outdated? Is there an overdependence on opinion articles and/or anecdotes? Are prior studies merely summarized, or are shortcomings discussed? Does the author indicate what is not known as well as what is?

c. Does the style seem appropriate for a research review? Does the review seem biased or laden with subjective opinions? Is there too little paraphrasing and too much quoting? Does the author use appropriately tentative language in describing the results of earlier studies?

2. Read the literature review section in one of the articles listed below. Critique the review, applying questions a through c from Question D.1 above.

- Artinian, N. T., & Duggan, C. H. (1993). Patterns of concerns and demands experienced by spouses following coronary artery bypass surgery. *Clinical Nursing Research, 2,* 278–295.
- Ganong, L. (1993). Nurses' perceptions of married and unmarried pregnant patients. *Western Journal of Nursing Research, 15,* 352–362.
- Janelli, L. M. (1993). Are there body image differences between older men and women? *Western Journal of Nursing Research, 15,* 327–339.
- Liehr, P., Todd, B., Rossi, M., & Culligan, M. (1992). Effect of venous support on edema and leg pain in patients after coronary artery bypass graft surgery. *Heart and Lung, 21,* 6–11.
- Mackey, M. C., & Stepans, M. E. F. (1994). Women's evaluation of their labor and delivery nurses. *Journal of Obstetric, Gynecologic, and Neonatal Nursing, 23,* 413–420.

E. *Special Projects*

1. Read the literature review section from a research article appearing in an issue of *Nursing Research* in the early 1980s (some possibilities are suggested below). Search the literature for more recent research on the topic of the article and update the review section. Don't forget to incorporate in your review the findings from the cited research article itself! Here are some possible articles:

   - Austin, J. K., McBride, A. B., & Davis, H. W. (1984). Parental attitude and adjustment to childhood epilepsy. *Nursing Research, 33,* 92–96.
   - Choi-Lao, A. (1981). Trace anesthetic vapors in hospital operating-room environments. *Nursing Research, 30,* 156–161.
   - Keane, A., Ducette, J., & Adler, D. (1985). Stress in ICU and non-ICU nurses. *Nursing Research, 34,* 231–236.
   - Newport, M. A. (1984). Conserving thermal energy and social integrity in the newborn. *Western Journal of Nursing Research, 6,* 175–188.
   - Schraeder, B. D., & Cooper, B. M. (1983). Development and temperament in very low birth weight infants. *Nursing Research, 32,* 331–335.

2. Select one of the problem statements from Question C.3. Conduct a literature search and identify 5 to 10 relevant references. Compare your references with those of your classmates in terms of relevance, recency, and type of information provided.

3. Read one of the studies suggested in Question D.2. Write a two-page summary of the research report, translating the information into everyday (i.e., nonresearch) language.

Chapter 5

CONCEPTUAL AND THEORETICAL CONTEXTS

A. *Matching Exercises*

1. Match each statement from Set B with one of the phrases in Set A. Indicate the letter corresponding to your response next to each of the statements in Set B.

SET A
a. Classic theory
b. Conceptual framework
c. Schematic model
d. Neither a, b, nor c
e. a, b, and c

SET B   **RESPONSE**
  1. Makes minimal use of language   _____
  2. Uses concepts as building blocks   _____
  3. Is essential in the conduct of good research   _____
  4. Can be used as a basis for generating hypotheses   _____
  5. Can be proved through empirical testing   _____
  6. Indicates a system of propositions that assert relationships
     among variables   _____
  7. Is developed inductively through observations   _____
  8. Consists of interrelated concepts organized in a rational
     scheme but does not specify formal relationships among the
     concepts   _____

9. Exists in nature and is awaiting scientific discovery   _____

10. May help to stimulate new directions in research   _____

2. Match each model from Set B with one of the nurse-theorists in Set A. Indicate the letter corresponding to your response next to each of the statements in Set B.

SET A

a. Orem
b. Pender
c. Levine
d. Parse
e. Rogers
f. Roy

SET B

1. Model of the Unitary Person   _____

2. Conservation Model   _____

3. Model of Man–Living–Health   _____

4. Model of Self-Care   _____

5. Adaptation Model   _____

6. Health Promotion Model   _____

B. Completion Exercises

Write the words or phrases that correctly complete the sentences below.

1. Theories are not found by scientists, they are _____

   _____ .

2. Deductions from theories are referred to as _____

   _____ .

3. Most of the conceptualizations of nursing practice would be called _____

   _____ .

4. Models attempt to represent reality with a minimal use of _____

   _____ .

5. $F = ma$ is an example of a(n) _____

   _____ .

6. In the statistical model $Y = \beta_1 X_1 + \beta_2 X_2 + e$, the βs are _____ _____ .

7. The four central concepts of conceptual models in nursing are _____ , _____ , _____ , and _____ .

8. The basic intellectual process underlying theory development is _____ _____ .

9. The acronym HBM stands for the _____ _____ .

10. Theoretical frameworks from nonnursing disciplines are sometimes referred to as _____ _____ .

C. Study Questions

1. Define the following terms. Compare your definition with the definition in the glossary or in Chapter 5 of the textbook.

   a. Descriptive theory: _____ _____ _____

   b. Macrotheory: _____ _____ _____

   c. Middle-range theory: _____ _____ _____

   d. Laws: _____ _____ _____

   e. Conceptual framework: _____

       _____

       _____

   f. Schematic model: _____

       _____

       _____

   g. Statistical model: _____

       _____

       _____

2. Read some recent issues of *Nursing Research* or another nursing research journal. Identify at least three different theories cited by nurse researchers in these research reports.
3. Using the statistical model presented in Chapter 5 of the textbook, suggest an alternative example for the Y (the dependent variable) and Xs the (independent variables). That is, hypothesize that some behavior or outcome of interest (Y) is due to the combined influence of four other factors (Xs).
4. Choose one of the conceptual frameworks of nursing that were described in this chapter. Develop a research hypothesis based on this framework.
5. Select one of the research questions listed in Section C from Chapter 3 of this Study Guide. Could your selected problem be developed within one of the nursing frameworks discussed in this chapter? Defend your answer.

D. Application Exercises

1. Valentine (1994)* developed a study derived from Rotter's social learning theory. Social learning theory postulates that human behaviors are contingent on the individual's expectancy that a particular behavior will be reinforced (rewarded). A key concept is locus of control, which is conceptualized as the degree to which a person perceives that rewards are a function of his or her own actions as opposed to external forces. Internal controllers are those who perceive themselves and their behavior as the major determinants of the reinforcement, while external controllers are those who tend to see little, if any, relationship between their own actions and subsequent reinforcement.

    Valentine hypothesized that individuals with an internal locus-of-control ori-

---

*This example is fictitious.

entation would be more likely to engage in preventive health care activities than those with an external orientation. As a rationale for this hypothesis, she reasoned that "internal" people see themselves as capable of controlling health outcomes, while externally oriented people see forces outside of their control as the major determinants of health outcomes; the "externals" are, therefore, less likely to engage in preventive health care behaviors. To test her hypothesis, Valentine operationalized "willingness to engage in preventive health care activities" as enrollment in a health maintenance organization (HMO) among a group of employees who were offered a choice between a traditional medical benefits package and HMO membership. Five hundred employees hired by a large industrial firm were administered a test that measured locus of control as part of the application process. Each new employee was offered a choice between the two medical programs. The 187 employees who chose HMO membership were found to have significantly higher (i.e., more internal) scores on the locus-of-control measure than the 313 employees who elected the traditional medical plan, thereby supporting Valentine's hypothesis.

Review and critique the above study, particularly with respect to its theoretical basis. To assist you in your critique, here are some guiding questions:

a. Examine the study variables. To what extent are they congruent with the conceptual perspective of the study's theoretical framework? Can you offer any suggestions for a different theoretical basis than the one used?

b. Do the hypotheses and research methods flow naturally from the theoretical framework, or does the link between them seem contrived?

c. In what way, if any, did the use of a theory enhance the value of this study? Compare the meaningfulness of the study as described with what it would have been had the same hypothesis been tested in the absence of a theory.

d. In what way, if any, did the outcome of the study affect the value of the theory? If the outcome had been different (e.g., no differences, or differences opposite to those predicted), what effect would that have had on the theory?

2. Read the introductory sections of one of the actual research studies cited below. Apply questions a through d from Question D.1 to one of these studies.

- Ahijevych, K., & Bernhard, L. (1994). Health-promoting behaviors of African American women. *Nursing Research, 43,* 86–89.
- Brown, S. J. (1992). Tailoring nursing care to the individual client: Empirical challenge of a theoretical concept. *Research in Nursing and Health, 15,* 39–46.
- Halm, M. A., et al. (1993). Behavioral responses of family members during critical illness. *Clinical Nursing Research, 2,* 414–437.
- Krausz, M., Kedem, P., Tal, Z., & Asmir, Y. (1992). Sex-role orientation and work adaptation of male nurses. *Research in Nursing and Health, 15,* 391–398.

- Lynam, L. E., & Miller, M. A. (1992). Mothers' and nurses' perceptions of the needs of women experiencing preterm labor. *Journal of Obstetric, Gynecologic, and Neonatal Nursing, 21,* 126–136.
- Mahon, N. E., Yarcheski, A., & Yarcheski, T. J. (1993). Health consequences of loneliness in adolescents. *Research in Nursing and Health, 16,* 23–31.
- Nyamathi, A., Jacoby, A., Constancia, P., & Ruvevich, S. (1992). Coping and adjustment of spouses of critically ill patients with cardiac disease. *Heart and Lung, 21,* 160–166.

E. Special Projects

1. One proposition of reinforcement theory is that *if* a behavior is rewarded (reinforced), *then* the behavior will be repeated (learned). Based on this theory and on your observation of behaviors in health settings or schools of nursing, suggest three nursing research problem statements.

2. Select one of the research questions in Table 3-2 of the textbook (or identify a research question of your own). Abstract a generalized issue (or several issues) from the statement. Search for an existing theory that might be applicable and appropriate.

3. Develop a researchable problem statement based on Pender's Health Promotion Model (Figure 5-1).

Chapter 6

THE ETHICAL CONTEXT OF NURSING RESEARCH

A. Matching Exercises

Match each of the descriptions in Set B with one of the procedures used to safeguard human subjects listed in Set A. Indicate the letter corresponding to the appropriate response next to each entry in Set B.

SET A
a. Freedom from harm or exploitation
b. Informed consent
c. Anonymity
d. Confidentiality

SET B   RESPONSE

1. A questionnaire distributed by mail bears an identification number in one corner. Respondents are assured their responses will not be individually divulged.   _____

2. Hospitalized children included in a study, and their parents, are told the aims and procedures of the research. Parents are asked to sign an authorization.   _____

3. Respondents in a questionnaire study in which the same respondents will be questioned twice are asked to place their own four-digit identification number on the questionnaire and to memorize the number. Respondents are assured their answers will remain private.   _____

4. Women who recently had a mastectomy are studied in terms of the psychological sequelae of the procedure. In the interview, sensitive questions are carefully worded. After the interview, debriefing with the respondent determines the need for psychological support.   _____

5. Women interviewed in the above study (number 4) are told that the information they provide will not be individually divulged.   _____

6. Subjects who volunteered for an experimental treatment for AIDS are warned of potential side effects and are asked to sign a waiver.   _____

7. After determining that a new intervention resulted in discomfort to subjects, the researcher discontinued the study.   _____

8. Unmarked questionnaires are distributed to a class of nursing students. The instructions indicate that the responses will not be individually divulged.   _____

9. The researcher assures subjects that they will be interviewed as part of the study at a single point in time and adheres to this promise.   _____

10. A questionnaire distributed to a sample of nursing students includes a statement indicating that completion and submission of the questionnaire will be construed as voluntary participation in a study, as fully described in an accompanying letter.   _____

B. Completion Exercises

Write the words or phrases that correctly complete the sentences below.

1. Ethical _____

   _____ arise when the rights of subjects and the demands of science are put into direct conflict.

2. One of the first internationally recognized efforts to establish ethical standards was the _____

   _____ .

3. The National Commission for the Protection of Human Subjects of Biomedical and Behavioral Research issued a well-known set of guidelines known as the

   _____

   _____ .

4. The most straightforward ethical precept is the protection of subjects from

   _____

   _____ .

5. Risks that are no greater than those ordinarily encountered in daily life are referred to as _____

   _____ .

6. The right to _____

   _____ means that prospective subjects have the right to voluntarily decide whether to participate in a study, without risk of penalty.

7. The researcher adheres to the principle of _____

   _____ by fully describing to subjects the nature of the study and the likely risks and benefits of participation.

8. When the researcher cannot link research information to the person who provided it, the condition known as _____

   _____ has prevailed.

9. Special procedures are often required to safeguard the rights of_____

   _____ subjects.

10. Committees established in institutions to review proposed research procedures with respect to their adherence to ethical guidelines are often called IRBs, or

    _____

    _____ .

C. Study Questions

1. Define the following terms. Compare your definition with the definition in Chapter 6 of the textbook or in the glossary.

a. Code of ethics: _____

_____

_____

b. Beneficence: _____

_____

_____

c. Debriefing: _____

_____

_____

d. Subject stipends: _____

_____

_____

e. Risk/benefit ratio: _____

_____

_____

f. Coercion: _____

_____

_____

g. Covert data collection: _____

_____

_____

h. Deception: _____

_____

_____

i. Confidentiality: _____

_____

_____

j. Informed consent: _____

_____

_____

k. Expedited review: _____

_____

_____

l. Vulnerable subjects: _____

_____

_____

2. Below are descriptions of several research studies. Suggest some ethical dilemmas that are likely to emerge for each.

a. A study of coping behaviors among rape victims _____

_____

_____

b. An unobtrusive observational study of fathers' behaviors in the delivery room

_____

_____

_____

c. An interview study of the antecedents of heroin addiction _____

_____

_____

d. A study of dependence among mentally retarded children _____

_____

_____

e. An investigation of the verbal interactions among schizophrenic patients __

_____

_____

f. A study of the effects of a new drug on human subjects _____

_____

_____

3. The following two studies involved the use of vulnerable subjects. Evaluate the ethical aspects of one or both of these studies, paying special attention to the manner in which the subjects' heightened vulnerability was handled.

- Archbold, P. G., Stewart, B. J., Greenlick, M. R., & Harvath, T. (1990). Mutuality and preparedness as predictors of caregiver role strain. *Research in Nursing and Health, 13,* 385–383.
- Nyamathi, A. M. (1991). Relationship of resources to emotional distress, somatic complaints, and high-risk behaviors in drug recovery and homeless minority women. *Research in Nursing and Health, 14,* 269–277.

4. In Chapter 6 in the textbook, two unethical studies were described (the study of syphilis among black men and the study in which live cancer cells were injected in elderly patients). Identify which ethical principles were transgressed in these studies.

5. A stipend of $5 was paid to the subjects who completed a questionnaire on breastfeeding in the following study:

- Hill, P. D. (1991). Predictors of breastfeeding duration among WIC and non-WIC mothers. *Public Health Nursing, 8,* 46–52.

   Read the introductory sections of the report and comment on the appropriateness of the stipend.

6. Comment on the risk/benefit ratio and other aspects of the following study, in which a mild form of deception was used:

- Forrester, D. A. (1990). AIDS-related risk factors, medical diagnosis, do-not-resusictate orders and aggressiveness of nursing care. *Nursing Research, 39,* 350–354.

D. Application Exercises

1. Kaye (1995)* investigated the behaviors of nursing students in crisis or emergency situations. The investigator was interested in comparing the behaviors of students from baccalaureate versus diploma programs to determine the adequacy of the preparation given to students in handling emergencies. Fifty students from both types of programs volunteered to participate in the study. The investigator wanted to observe reactions to crises as they might occur naturally, so the participants were not told the exact nature of the study. Each student was instructed to take the vital signs of a "patient," purportedly to evaluate the students' skills. The "patient," who was described as another student but who in fact was a confederate of the investigator, simulated an epileptic seizure while the vital signs were being taken. A research assistant, who was unaware of the purpose of the study and who did not know the educational background of the subjects, observed the

*This study is fictitious.

timeliness and appropriateness of the students' responses to the situation through a one-way mirror. Subjects were not required to fill out any forms that recorded their identities. Immediately after participation, subjects were debriefed as to the true nature of the study and were paid a $10 stipend.

Consider the aspects of this study in terms of the issues discussed in this chapter. To assist you in your review, here are some guiding questions:

a. Were the subjects in this study at risk of physical or psychological harm? Were they at risk of exploitation?

b. Did the subjects in the study derive any benefits from their participation? Did the nursing community or society at large benefit? How would you assess the risk/benefit ratio?

c. Were the subjects' rights to self-determination violated? Was there any coercion involved? Was full disclosure made to subjects before participation? Was informed consent given to subjects and documented?

d. Were subjects treated fairly? Was their right to privacy protected?

e. What ethical dilemmas does this study present? How, if at all, can the dilemmas be resolved? To what extent *were* they resolved?

f. What type of human subjects review would be appropriate for a study such as the one described?

2. Read one or more of the articles listed below. Respond to questions a through f from Question D.1 in terms of these actual research studies.

- Algase, D. L. (1992). Cognitive discriminants of wandering among nursing home residents. *Nursing Research, 41,* 78–81.

- Damrosch, S., & Scholler-Jaquish, A. (1993). Nurses' experiences with impaired nurse co-workers. *Applied Nursing Research, 6,* 154–160.

- McCain, G. C., & Deatrick, J. A. (1994). The experience of high-risk pregnancy. *Journal of Obstetric, Gynecologic, and Neonatal Nursing, 23,* 421–428.

- Rodriguez-Fisher, L., Bourguignon, C., & Good, B. V. (1993). Dietary fiber nursing intervention. *Clinical Nursing Research, 2,* 464–477.

- Schumacher, K. L., Dodd, M. J., & Paul, S. M. (1993). The stress process in family caregivers of persons receiving chemotherapy. *Research in Nursing and Health, 16,* 395–404.

E. Special Projects

1. Prepare a brief summary of a hypothetical study in which there are at least three major benefits to subjects participating in the study.

2. Prepare a brief summary of a hypothetical study in which the costs and benefits are both high. When the costs and benefits are essentially balanced, how should the researcher decide whether or not to proceed?

3. Skim the following research report, and draft an informed consent form for this study:

   • Sampselle, C. M., & DeLancey, J. O. L. (1992). The urine stream interruption test and pelvic muscle function. *Nursing Research, 41,* 73–77.

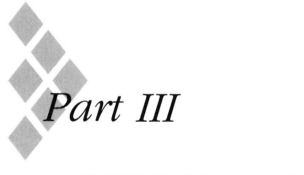

Part III

DESIGNS FOR NURSING RESEARCH

Chapter 7

SELECTING A
RESEARCH DESIGN

A. Matching Exercises

Match each research question from Set B with a phrase from Set A that indicates the nature of the comparison implied in the research question. Indicate the letter corresponding to your response next to each statement in Set B.

SET A

a. Comparison of two or more groups
b. Comparison of a group at two or more points in time
c. Comparison of a group under different circumstances
d. Comparison of relative rankings

SET B   **RESPONSE**

1. Is morale among the institutionalized elderly related to their self-care abilities?   _____

2. Do married and unmarried pregnant women differ in their perceptions of nursing care after delivery?   _____

3. Do women instructed in the benefits of breast self-examination (BSE) increase the frequency of BSE?   _____

4. Do men and women have different styles of coping after the death of a spouse?   _____

5. Do patients give different oral temperature readings immediately after they have ingested iced water compared with when no iced water is ingested?   _____

6. Is hospital noise intensity related to patients' amount of time spent in rapid-eye movement (REM) sleep?   _____

7. Are women who run regularly more likely than nonrunners to develop amenorrhea?   _____

8. Does the level of maternal attachment among pregnant women change after they have seen a sonogram image of their fetus?   _____

9. Are there fewer complaints from patients on days when they are fed breakfast at 8:00 AM than on days when they are fed breakfast at 7:00 AM?   _____

10. Are there differences in the levels of depression among U.S. immigrants from Central America, Asia, and Europe?   _____

B. Completion Exercises

Write the words or phrases that correctly complete the sentences below.

1. The aspect of research design that concerns whether or not there is an intervention involves the distinction between _____ and _____ designs.

2. Researchers generally design their studies to include one or more type of _____ _____ to make their results more interpretable.

3. Highly structured and contrived settings designed specifically for the conduct of research are known as _____ _____ settings.

4. Most in-depth qualitative studies occur in _____ _____ settings.

5. Designs for qualitative studies tend to be highly _____ _____ .

6. When data are collected at a single point in time, the design is referred to as _____ .

7. Longitudinal studies conducted to determine the long-term outcome of some condition or intervention are called _____

   _____ .

8. Studies that combine features of a cohort study with a cross-sectional study are using the design known as _____

   _____ .

9. A prospective design is more rigorous in elucidating casual relationships than a(n) _____

   _____ design.

10. Any influence that can distort the results of the study is known as a(n)_____

    _____ .

11. A design that maximizes the variability in the dependent variable that can be attributed to the independent variable is enhancing the _____

    _____ of the study.

12. When comparison groups are designed to be as different as possible, the_____

    _____ of

    the design is enhanced.

C. Study Questions

1. Define the following terms. Compare your definition with the definition in Chapter 7 of the textbook or in the glossary.

   a. Research design: _____

      _____

      _____

   b. Intervention: _____

      _____

      _____

   c. Unstructured research design: _____

   _____

   _____

   d. Cross-sectional design: _____

   _____

   _____

   e. Longitudinal design: _____

   _____

   _____

   f. Trend study: _____

   _____

   _____

   g. Panel study: _____

   _____

   _____

   h. Attrition: _____

   _____

   _____

   i. Double-blind procedures: _____

   _____

   _____

   j. Retrospective design: _____

   _____

   _____

   k. Prospective design: _____

   _____

   _____

2. Suppose you wanted to study self-esteem among successful dieters who lost 20 or more pounds and maintained their weight loss for at least 6 months. Specify at least two different types of comparison strategies that would provide a useful comparative context for this study.

3. Fawcett and Weiss, cited below, conducted a study of women's adaptation to cesarean delivery and collected the data for their study while the women were still in the hospital. Review the study and consider how the research setting might influence the findings. What might be the drawbacks of conducting the study in an alternative setting?

   • Fawcett, J., & Weiss, M. E. (1993). Cross-cultural adaptation to cesarean birth. *Western Journal of Nursing Research, 15,* 282–297.

4. Suppose you wanted to study the coping strategies of AIDS patients at different points in the progress of the disease. Design a cross-sectional study to research this question, describing how subjects would be selected. Now design a longitudinal study to research the same problem. Identify the strengths and weaknesses of the two approaches.

5. Suppose that you were interested in testing the hypothesis that the use of IUDs could cause infertility. Describe how such a hypothesis could be tested using a retrospective design. Now describe a prospective design for the same study. Compare the strengths and weaknesses of the two approaches.

D. *Application Exercises*

1. Roicke (1995)* hypothesized that aging negatively affects intellectual capacity and motor responsivity. To test this hypothesis, she randomly selected the names of 250 men aged 70 years or older; 250 men in their 50s; and 250 men in their 30s from the residents living in a mid-sized city in Illinois. Roicke realized that intellectual capacity is sometimes correlated with social class. Furthermore, mortality rates vary by social class. Therefore, the subjects were selected in such a way that half in each group were from lower-income households (annual household incomes of $25,000 or less) and half were from higher-income households (annual household incomes over $25,000). The basic design for the analysis, therefore, was as follows:

	AGE GROUP		
INCOME GROUP	30s	50s	70s
≤ $25,000			
> $25,000			

   The 750 individuals were administered an individual intelligence test that measured verbal aptitude, problem solving, quantitative skills, spatial aptitude,

*This example is fictitious.

and overall intelligence. In addition, the participants were given various reaction-time tests. The analysis of the data revealed that, as hypothesized, intelligence declined with age in both income groups. Except on the measure of verbal aptitude, the subjects in their 30s scored highest, and the subjects in their 70s scored lowest on the subtests of intellectual capacity and on overall intelligence. The same pattern was observed for reaction time. Roicke concluded that the aging process causes deterioration of both intellectual and motor capacity.

Review and critique Roicke's study. Suggest alternative designs or other modifications for testing the researcher's hypothesis. To assist you in your critique, here are some guiding questions:

a. Is this design cross-sectional or longitudinal?

b. What problems, if any, does this design pose in terms of testing the hypothesis? What design, if any, might be more appropriate? What difficulties, if any, would the researcher have had in implementing your recommended design?

c. What extraneous variables did the researcher identify, and how were they controlled? How did this affect the precision of the design?

d. What extraneous variables do you think should have been controlled but were not? Why might the researcher have decided not to control these variables?

2. Below are several suggested research articles. Read the introductory and methods sections of one or more of these articles, and respond to the questions in Exercise D.1 in terms of these actual research studies.

• Beach, E. K., Maloney, B. H., Plocica, A. R., Sherry, S. E., Weaver, M., Luthringer, L., & Utz, S. (1992). The spouse: A factor in recovery after acute myocardial infarction. *Heart and Lung, 21,* 30–38.

• Heidrich, S. M. (1993). The relationship between physical health and psychological well-being in elderly women: A developmental perspective. *Research in Nursing and Health, 16,* 123–130.

• Polivka, B. J., Nickel, J. T., & Wilkins, J. R. (1993). Cerebral palsy: Evaluation of a model of risk. *Research in Nursing and Health, 16,* 113–122.

• Walker, L. O., & Montgomery, E. (1994). Maternal identity and role attainment: Long-term relations to children's development. *Nursing Research, 43,* 105–110.

E. Special Projects

1. Suppose that you wanted to compare premature and normal babies in terms of their development at 5 years of age. Describe a broad design for such a study, being careful to indicate the number of times data would be collected. Discuss the rationale for your design.

2. A nurse researcher is interested in testing the effect of packing sugar on a wound on the wound-healing process. Describe a design you would recommend for this problem, being careful to indicate what extraneous variables you would need to control and how you would control them, and what comparisons could be made to enhance the interpretability of the results. Discuss the rationale for your decisions.

3. Chapter 7 identified four types of situations in which it might be appropriate to use multiple points of data collection. Develop a researchable problem statement for each of these four situations. Develop a design for studying one or more of these problems.

   a. Time-related phenomena: _____

   _____

   _____

   b. Time-sequenced phenomena: _____

   _____

   _____

   c. Comparative purposes: _____

   _____

   _____

   d. Enhancement of research control: _____

   _____

   _____

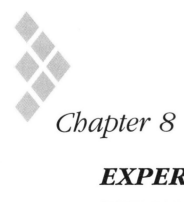

Chapter 8

EXPERIMENTAL, QUASI-EXPERIMENTAL, AND NONEXPERIMENTAL DESIGNS

A. Matching Exercises

1. Match each design representation from Set B with one of the design types from Set A. Indicate the letter corresponding to your response next to each item in Set B.

SET A

a. True experimental design
b. Quasi-experimental design
c. Pre-experimental design
d. Nonexperimental design

SET B   **RESPONSE**

1. $\underline{\quad X \quad O \quad}$

    $\qquad O$ _____

2. $O_1O_2O_3O_4 \quad X \quad O_5O_6O_7O_8$ _____

3. $\underline{R \quad X \quad O}$

    $R \qquad O$ _____

4. $\underline{O_1 \quad X \quad O_2}$

    $O_1 \qquad O_1$ _____

5. O_1 X O_2 _____

6. $\underline{R \quad X_1 \quad O}$
     $\underline{R \quad X_2 \quad O}$
     $R \qquad\quad O$ _____

7. $\underline{O_1 \qquad\quad O_2}$
     $O_1 \qquad\quad O_2$ _____

8. $\underline{O_1 O_2 O_3 O_4 \quad X \quad O_5 O_6 O_7 O_8}$
     $O_1 O_2 O_3 O_4 \quad X \quad O_5 O_6 O_7 O_8$ _____

2. Match each problem statement from Set B with one (or more) of the phrases from Set A that indicates a potential reason for using a nonexperimental approach. Indicate the letter(s) corresponding to your response next to each statement in Set B.

SET A

a. Independent variable cannot be manipulated
b. Ethical constraints on manipulation
c. Practical constraints on manipulation
d. No constraints on manipulation

SET B

1. Does the use of certain tampons cause toxic shock syndrome?   _____

2. Does heroin addiction among mothers affect Apgar scores of infants?   _____

3. Is the age of a hemodialysis patient related to the incidence of the disequilibrium syndrome?   _____

4. What body positions aid respiratory function?   _____

5. Does the ingestion of saccharin cause cancer in humans?   _____

6. Does a nurse's attitude toward the elderly affect his or her choice of a clinical specialty?   _____

7. Does the use of touch by nursing staff affect patient morale?   _____

8. Does a nurse's gender affect his or her salary and rate of promotion?   _____

9. Does extreme athletic exertion in young women cause amenorrhea?   _____

10. Does assertiveness training affect a psychiatric nurse's job performance?   _____

B. Completion Exercises

Write the words or phrases that correctly complete the sentences below.

1. In an experiment, the researcher manipulates the _____

   _____ variable.

2. The manipulation that the researcher introduces is referred to as the experimental

   _____

   _____ .

3. Randomization is performed so that groups will be formed without _____

   _____ .

4. Another term for randomization is _____

   _____ .

5. When more than one independent variable is being simultaneously manipulated

   by the researcher, the design is referred to as a(n) _____

   _____ .

6. The most typical method of randomization is through the use of a(n) _____

   _____ .

7. When data are gathered before the institution of some treatment, the initial data

   gathering is referred to as the _____

   _____ .

8. When neither the subjects nor the individuals collecting data know in which

   group a subject is participating, the procedures are called _____

   _____ .

9. Each factor in an experimental design must have two or more _____

   _____ .

10. Another term used for a repeated measures design is a(n) _____

    _____ design.

11. A primary objective of a true experiment is to enable the researcher to infer

    _____

    _____ .

12. When a true experimental design is not used, the control group is usually referred to as the _____ _____ group.

13. A research design that lacks the controls of a quasi-experiment is referred to as a(n) _____ _____ design.

14. A quasi-experimental design that involves repeated observations over time is referred to as the _____ _____ .

15. The difficulty with a nonequivalent control group design is that the experimental and comparison groups cannot be assumed to be _____ _____ before the intervention.

16. When no variable is manipulated in a study, the research is called _____ _____ .

17. Ex post facto research is also referred to as _____ _____ research.

18. Correlation does not prove _____ _____ .

19. A retrospective design that involves a comparison of a group with a specified disease or condition with another group without the disease or condition is called a(n) _____ _____ design.

20. The fallacy of "post hoc ergo propter" lies in an assumption that one thing caused another simply because the presumed cause _____ _____ the presumed effect.

C. Study Questions

1. Define the following terms. Compare your definition with the definition in the glossary or in Chapter 8 of the textbook.

a. Experiment: _____

_____

_____

b. Manipulation: _____

_____

_____

c. Randomization: _____

_____

_____

d. Control group: _____

_____

_____

e. Clinical trial: _____

_____

_____

f. Solomon four-group design: _____

_____

_____

g. Interaction effects: _____

_____

_____

h. Cluster randomization: _____

_____

_____

i. Hawthorne effect: _____

_____

_____

j. Quasi-experiment: _____

_____

_____

k. Rival hypothesis: _____

_____

_____

l. Ex post facto research: _____

_____

_____

m. Univariate descriptive study: _____

_____

_____

n. Self-selection: _____

_____

_____

2. Below are 20 subjects who have volunteered for a study of the effects of noise on pulse rate. Ten must be assigned to the low-volume group and 10 to a high-volume group. Use the table of random numbers in Table 8-1 of the text to randomly assign subjects to groups and groups to treatments.

J. Foster	S. Dunne
M. Higley	W. Niro
J. Enright	B. Hakan
D. Rutherford	B. Schwing
L. Kuharek	J. Traetta
C. Prodromos	P. Moss
J. Kurz	R. Phelps
C. Paganelli	E. Stautner
A. Schwab	J. Trice
J. Lamphier	M. Hohensee

3. Assume all the subjects in the first column above are in their 20s and all the subjects in the second column are in their 30s. How good a job did your randomization do in terms of equalizing the experimental and control groups according to age? Add 10 more names to each age group and assign these additional 20 subjects. Now compare the low-volume and high-volume groups in terms of the age distribution. Did doubling the sample size improve the distribution of the subjects' ages within the two volume-level groups?

4. Read one of the articles listed under Substantive References in Chapter 8 of the textbook. Using the notation presented in Figures 8-4 through 8-13, diagram the research design of the study.

5. A nurse researcher found a relationship between teenagers' level of knowledge about birth control and their level of sexual activity. That is, teenagers with higher levels of sexual activity knew more about birth control than teenagers with less sexual activity. Suggest at least three interpretations for this finding.

a. _____

_____

_____

b. _____

_____

_____

c. _____

_____

_____

6. Does Exercise C.5 describe a research problem that is *inherently* nonexperimental? Why or why not?

7. Indicate which of the following variables *inherently* can or cannot be manipulated by a researcher.*

a. Age at onset of obesity _____

b. Amount of auditory stimulation _____

c. Number of cigarettes smoked _____

d. Infant's birthweight _____

e. Blood type _____

f. Preoperative anxiety _____

g. Type of nursing curriculum _____

h. Attitudes toward nurses' extended role _____

i. Nurses' shift assignments _____

*Remember that *manipulation* does not refer to whether or not the variable can be *affected* by a researcher; it refers to the researcher's ability to randomly assign individuals to different levels of the variable or to different groups.

    j. Type of birth control method used _____

    k. Mother–infant bonding _____

    l. Use of atrioventricular shunt versus atrioventricular fistula _____

    m. Fluid intake _____

    n. Morale of dying patients' family members _____

    o. Nurses' fringe benefits _____

8. Refer to the 10 hypotheses in Exercises C.5 and C.6 of Chapter 3. Indicate below whether these hypotheses could be tested using an experimental/quasi-experimental approach, a nonexperimental approach, or both.

	EXPERIMENTAL/ QUASI-EXPERIMENTAL	NONEXPERIMENTAL	BOTH
5a	_____	_____	_____
5b	_____	_____	_____
5c	_____	_____	_____
5d	_____	_____	_____
5e	_____	_____	_____
6a	_____	_____	_____
6b	_____	_____	_____
6c	_____	_____	_____
6d	_____	_____	_____
6e	_____	_____	_____

9. Can most problems that are researched using an experimental approach be researched using a nonexperimental approach? How about vice versa? Why or why not?

10. In the following study, the researchers conducted a double-blind experiment. Review the design for this study, and comment on the appropriateness of the double-blind procedures. What biases were the researchers trying to avoid? Were they successful?

    • Simms, S. G., Rhodes, V. A., & Madsen, R. W. (1993). Comparison of prochlorperazine and lorazepam antiemetic regimens in the control of post-chemotherapy symptoms. *Nursing Research, 42,* 234–239.

D. Application Exercises

1. Kirkpatrick (1994)† wanted to test the effectiveness of a new relaxation/biofeedback intervention on menopause symptoms. She invited women who presented themselves in an outpatient clinic with complaints of severe hot flashes to participate in the study of the experimental treatment. These 30 women were asked to record, every day for 1 week before their treatment, the frequency and duration of their hot flashes. During the intervention, which involved six 1-hour sessions over a 3-week period, the women again recorded their symptoms. Then, 4 weeks after the treatment, the women were asked to record their hot flashes over a 5-day period. At the end of the study, Kirkpatrick found that both the frequency and average duration of the hot flashes had been significantly reduced in this sample of women. She concluded that her new treatment was an effective alternative to estrogen replacement therapy in treating menopausal hot flashes.

   Review and critique this study. Suggest alternative designs for testing the effectiveness of the treatment. To assist you in your critique, here are some guiding questions:

   a. Is the design described above experimental, quasi-experimental, or pre-experimental? Diagram the design using the notation shown in Figures 8-4 through 8-13 of the text.

   b. The investigator concluded that the outcome (i.e., the reduction in the frequency and duration of the women's hot flashes) was attributable to the experimental treatment. Can you offer one or more alternative explanations to account for the outcome? Discuss the inference of causality in the context of this research design.

   c. Consider your responses to part b above. If you have identified any weaknesses in the design of this research, suggest a modified design that would improve the study. In what way does your new design eliminate the problems of the original design?

2. Below are several suggested research articles. Read one or more of these articles, and respond to questions a through c from Question D.1 in terms of these actual research studies.

   • Boehm, S., Schlenk, E. A., Raleigh, E., & Ronis, D. (1993). Behavioral analysis and behavioral strategies to improve self-management of Type II diabetes. *Clinical Nursing Research, 2,* 327–344.

   • Day, R. A., Arnaud, S. S., & Monsma, M. (1993). Effectiveness of a handwashing program. *Clinical Nursing Research, 2,* 24–40.

---

†This example is fictitious.

- Erler, C. J., & Rudman, S. D. (1993). Effect of intensive care simulation on anxiety of nursing students in the clinical ICU. *Heart and Lung, 22,* 259–265.

- Grant, L. P., Wanger, L. I., & Neill, K. M. (1994). Fiber-fortified feedings in immobile patients. *Clinical Nursing Research, 3,* 166–172.

- Liehr, P., Todd, B., Rossi, M., & Culligan, M. (1992). Effect of venous support on edema and leg pain in patients after coronary artery bypass graft surgery. *Heart and Lung, 21,* 6–11.

3. Grey (1995)‡ hypothesized that the absence of socioemotional supports among the elderly results in a high level of chronic health problems and low morale. She tested this hypothesis by interviewing a sample of 250 residents of one community who were aged 65 years and older. The respondents were randomly selected from a list of town residents. Grey used several measures regarding the availability of socioemotional supports: (1) whether the respondent lived with any kin; (2) whether the respondent had any living children who resided within 30 minutes away; (3) the total number of interactions the respondent had had in the previous week with kin not residing in his or her household; and (4) the number of close friends in whom the respondent felt he or she could confide. Based on responses to the various questions on social support, respondents were classified in one of three groups: low social support, moderate social support, and high social support.

   In a 6-month follow-up interview, Grey collected information from 214 respondents about the frequency and intensity of the respondents' illnesses in the preceding 6-months, their hospitalization record, their overall satisfaction with life, and their attitudes toward their own aging. An analysis of the data revealed that the low-support group had significantly more health problems, lower life satisfaction ratings, and lower acceptance of their aging than the other two groups. Grey concluded that the availability of social supports resulted in better physical and mental adjustment to old age.

   Review and critique this study. Suggest alternative designs for testing the researcher's hypothesis. To assist you in your critique, here are some guiding questions:

   a. Is this research nonexperimental? If so, is it *inherently* nonexperimental? Why or why not? If so, what *type* of nonexperimental research is it?

   b. Examine the criteria for causality presented in Chapter 8 of the text. Does this study meet all the criteria for establishing causality?

   c. The researcher concluded that her independent variable (amount of social support) "caused" certain outcomes (mental and physical health status in the

---

‡This example is fictitious.

elderly). Can you offer two or more alternative explanations to account for the outcome?

d. Consider your responses to parts b and c above. If you have identified any weaknesses in the design of this research, suggest modifications that would improve the study design.

4. Below are several suggested research articles. Read the introductory and methods sections of one or more of these articles, and respond to questions a through d from Question D.3 in terms of these actual research studies.

- Broom, B. L. (1994). Impact of marital quality and psychological well-being on parental sensitivity. *Nursing Research, 43,* 138–143.
- Hamilton, G. A., & Seidman, R. N. (1993). A comparison of the recovery period for women and men after an acute myocardial infarction. *Heart and Lung, 22,* 308–315.
- LaMontagne, L. L., Hepworth, J. T., Johnson, B. D., & Deshpande, J. K. (1994). Psychophysiological responses of parents to pediatric critical care stress. *Clinical Nursing Research, 3,* 104–118.
- Monsen, R. B. (1992). Autonomy, coping, and self-care agency in healthy adolescents and in adolescents with spina bifida. *Journal of Pediatric Nursing, 7,* 9–13.
- Polk-Walker, G. C., Chan, W., Meltzer, A. A., Goldapp, G., & Williams, B. (1993). Psychiatric recidivism prediction factors. *Western Journal of Nursing Research, 15,* 163–173.

E. Special Projects

1. Suppose that you were interested in testing the hypothesis that a regular regimen of exercise reduces blood pressure, improves cardiovascular efficiency, and increases coronary circulation. Design a quasi-experiment to test the hypothesis. Evaluate this design in terms of the ability to make causal inferences. Design a true experiment to test the same hypothesis, and compare the kinds of conclusions that can be drawn with this design with those from the quasi-experiment. Describe how you might design an ex post facto study to test the same hypothesis.

2. Generate a hypothesis of your own in which the aim is to establish a cause-and-effect relationship. Design both a quasi-experiment and a true experiment, and compare how the designs address possible alternative explanations of the results.

3. Suppose that you were interested in testing the hypothesis that the use of IUDs could cause infertility. Describe how such a hypothesis could be tested using a retrospective design. Now describe a prospective design for the same study. Compare the strengths and weaknesses of the two approaches. Could an experimental or quasi-experimental design be used? Why or why not?

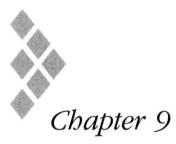

Chapter 9

ADDITIONAL TYPES
OF RESEARCH

A. Matching Exercises

Match each problem statement from Set B with one (or more) of the types of research that could be undertaken to address the problem listed in Set A. Indicate the letter(s) corresponding to your response next to each of the statements in Set B.

SET A
a. Survey research
b. Field research
c. Evaluation research
d. Needs assessment
e. Historical research
f. Case study
g. Methodological research

SET B   **RESPONSE**

1. What types of social and health services are needed by the rural elderly?   _____

2. Does the assurance of anonymity to respondents increase self-reports of socially undesirable behavior such as child or spouse abuse?   _____

3. Do parents approve of sex education in the schools?   _____

4. Can a new curriculum improve students' scores on the licen-

Polit DF, Hungler BP: STUDY GUIDE FOR NURSING RESEARCH:
PRINCIPLES AND METHODS, 5th ed. © 1995 J.B. Lippincott Company.

sure examination at the Eastern University's School of Nursing?   _____

5. What is the effect of social change regarding men's and women's roles on the image of male nurses?   _____

6. Are patients' ratings of nurses' job performance less accurate than supervisors' ratings?   _____

7. Is a radio-based media campaign more effective than a print-based media campaign in recruiting blood donors?   _____

8. How does a community react to the stress of a natural disaster such as a hurricane?   _____

9. How do nursing faculty feel about the inclusion of nursing research courses in the undergraduate curriculum?   _____

10. Does the block rotation method of scheduling result in a lower absentee rate among nursing staff than a random rotation method?   _____

B. Completion Exercises

Write the words or phrases that correctly complete the sentences below.

1. Surveys rarely involve questioning an entire _____
_____ , but rely instead on samples.

2. Interviews using the _____
_____ are less expensive than in-person interviews.

3. When a survey instrument is self-administered, it is referred to as a(n) _____
_____ .

4. In evaluation research, behavioral objectives should focus on the behavior of the
_____
_____ of a program, not the agents.

5. Program evaluations that do not focus exclusively on intended outcomes but that consider broader, unintended ones as well are often referred to as _____
_____ .

6. Evaluations that focus on the net effects of an intervention are referred to as

_____

_____ .

7. A(n) _____

_____ is a form of evaluation undertaken to determine the financial effects of a

program.

8. The method of collecting needs assessment data by questioning knowledgeable

individuals is known as the _____

_____ .

9. Secondary analysis involves the use of previously collected _____

_____ .

10. When a researcher analyzes data as a secondary analysis and either aggregates or

disaggregates the data differently than in the original research, we say that there

has been a change in the _____

_____ .

11. In meta-analyses, the index that is calculated for each study to summarize the

magnitude of group differences is the _____

_____ .

12. Respondents in a Delphi study are referred to as a(n) _____

_____ .

13. Methodological research is so named because it is research conducted for the

purpose of developing or refining research _____

_____ .

14. In content analysis, the most common units of analysis used by nurse researchers

are _____ and _____

_____ .

15. Studies of individuals in naturalistic social settings are referred to as _____

_____ .

16. Ethnographic research focuses on human _____

    _____ .

17. Phenomenological research focuses on the _____

    _____ of phenomena as experienced

    by people.

18. The disciplinary roots of ethnography is _____; of phe-

    nomenology is _____; and of ethnomethodology is ____

    _____ .

19. In historical research, first-hand accounts of events or experiences are referred to

    as _____

    _____ .

20. Historical researchers who question the authenticity of a document or artifact are

    invoking _____

    _____ criticism.

C. Study Questions

1. Define the following terms. Compare your definition with the definition in Chapter 9 of the textbook or in the glossary.

    a. Survey research: _____

    _____

    _____

    b. Personal interview: _____

    _____

    _____

    c. Census: _____

    _____

    _____

d. Evaluation research: _____

_____

_____

e. Process evaluation: _____

_____

_____

f. Summative evaluation: _____

_____

_____

g. Net impact: _____

_____

_____

h. Policy research: _____

_____

_____

i. Needs assessment: _____

_____

_____

j. Indicators approach: _____

_____

_____

k. Secondary analysis: _____

_____

_____

l. Meta-analysis: _____

_____

_____

m. Methodological research: _____

_____

_____

n. Ethnonursing research: _____

_____

_____

o. Historical research: _____

_____

_____

p. Case study: _____

_____

_____

2. Suppose that you were interested in studying the problems below by means of a survey. For each, indicate whether you would recommend using a personal interview, a telephone interview, or a questionnaire to collect the data. Justify your response.

a. How well informed are nursing students about venereal disease? _____

_____

_____

b. What are the coping strategies and behaviors of newly widowed individuals?

_____

_____

_____

c. What is the attitude of the general population toward health maintenance organizations? _____

_____

_____

d. What are the emotional sequelae of having an organ transplantation? _____

_____

_____

e. Do nursing faculty in different clinical specialties differ in their scholarly productivity? _____

_____

_____

f. Are nurses' attitudes toward unionization related to their incomes? _____

_____

_____

g. Are the rural elderly more socially isolated than the urban elderly? _____

_____

_____

h. Are people's attitudes toward in vitro fertilization related to their religious affiliation? _____

_____

_____

i. Is the socialization process for new nursing graduates in their first job smoother in large or small hospitals? _____

_____

_____

j. What type of nursing communications do presurgical patients find most helpful? _____

_____

_____

3. Listed below are several programs or policies that could be evaluated. For each, think of one or more objectives that such a program might have that would be amenable to evaluation, and state them as *behavioral* objectives. Remember that it is the intended behavior of *recipients* that must be specified.

a. A continuing education workshop on new techniques in monitoring intra-cranial pressure
b. A seminar to improve nurses' instructions to dialysis patients regarding the hygienic care of their shunts
c. A crisis intervention program for rape victims
d. Procedures to educate primaparas with regard to breastfeeding their infants
e. An instructional unit that teaches techniques in respiratory assessment to nursing students.

4. Below are several research problems. Indicate for each whether you think the problem should be studied using a survey approach or a field study approach. Justify your response.

    a. By what process do new nursing home residents learn to adapt to their environments?

    b. What aspects of their jobs are related to job satisfaction among school nurses?

    c. What is the relationship between a teenager's health-risk appraisal and various forms of risk-taking behavior (e.g., smoking, sexual activity without contraception, using drugs, etc.)?

    d. What aspects of the lifestyles of urban disadvantaged women place them at especially high risk of pregnancy and childbirth complications?

    e. How are the dynamics of nurse–patient interaction affected by the presence of a physician?

5. A nurse researcher is developing a study to evaluate the effectiveness of a program that uses nurse practitioners to manage common respiratory infections. Suggest a design for an impact analysis.

6. Consider a client group of interest to you. Suggest an approach for conducting a needs assessment for this group.

7. Read the methodological study by Savedra and her colleagues (1993) in *Nursing Research,* volume 42, pages 5–9. Design at least one substantive study that would use their measure of pain assessment in children as the dependent variable.

8. Suppose you were interested in conducting a case study on a person with insomnia. Describe what your approach would be. What types of data would you collect? What might be some of the ethical considerations of such a study?

D. Application Exercises

1. Furey (1994)* studied the contraceptive practices of university students at three large Midwestern universities. In addition to obtaining descriptive information, he wanted to test the hypothesis that students who report favorable experiences with health care personnel relating to contraceptives are more likely than those with unfavorable experiences to practice birth control effectively. A random sample of 500 students from each university was sent a mailed questionnaire. A total of 715 usable questionnaires were returned.

    The questionnaire included questions on sexual experience, contraceptive use history, perceived ease of access to birth control, feelings about seeking out contraceptive information, knowledge of on-campus contraceptive services, and experiences with health care personnel related to contraceptives. The questionnaire also asked about the student's age, ethnicity, year in college, major, father's occupation, marital status, religion, and grade point average.

    Furey's data revealed that while most students were sexually experienced,

*This example is fictitious.

fewer than half had used any birth control during their last intercourse. About 60% of the sexually active students had had a contact with health care personnel relating to contraceptives, and of these, 70% described their experience in positive terms. In comparing those who had had favorable and unfavorable experiences, Furey found that a significantly higher percentage of those with a favorable experience (68% versus 42%) had used some form of contraceptive at last intercourse. He concluded that a favorable experience with health care personnel leads to better contraceptive utilization. He speculated that those with more positive experiences were better informed about and more accepting of contraception than those with negative experiences and hence practiced birth control more conscientiously.

Review and critique this study. Suggest alternative methods for conducting this research. To assist you in your critique, here are some guiding questions:

a. Is this research nonexperimental? If so, is it *inherently* nonexperimental? Why or why not?

b. What type of research study is this, in terms of the types discussed in this chapter? Could the same research problem be studied using an alternative approach (i.e., one of the other types of research discussed in the chapter)?

c. Examine the criteria for causality presented in Chapter 8 of the text. Does this study meet all the criteria for establishing causality?

d. The researcher concluded that the independent variable (quality of the students' experience with health care personnel) "caused" a certain outcome (contraceptive utilization). Can you offer alternative explanations to account for the outcome?

e. Consider your responses to parts b and c, above. If you have identified any weaknesses in the design of this research, suggest modifications that would improve the study design.

f. Prepare two or three hypotheses that you could test in a secondary analysis of this researcher's data.

2. Below are several suggested research articles. Skim one or more of these articles and respond to questions a through f from Question D.1 in terms of this actual research study.

- Nicholas, P. K., & Webster, A. (1993). Hardiness and social support in human immunodeficiency virus. *Applied Nursing Research, 6,* 132–135.

- O'Brien, M. T. (1993). Multiple sclerosis: The role of social support and disability. *Clinical Nursing Research, 2,* 67–85.

- Okrainec, G. D. (1994). Perceptions of nursing education held by male nursing students. *Western Journal of Nursing Research, 16,* 94–107.

- Ornitz, A. W., & Brown, M. A. (1993). Family coping and premenstrual symptomatology. *Journal of Obstetric, Gynecologic, and Neonatal Nursing, 22,* 49–55.

- Woods, N. F., Taylor, D., Mitchell, E. S., & Lentz, M. J. (1992). Perimenstrual symptoms and health-seeking behavior. *Western Journal of Nursing Research, 14,* 418–443.

E. Special Projects

1. Generate one problem statement for each of the following types of research that were described in this chapter.

   a. Survey research: _____

   _____

   _____

   b. Evaluation research: _____

   _____

   _____

   c. Needs assessment: _____

   _____

   _____

   d. Ethnographic research: _____

   _____

   _____

   e. Phenomenologic research: _____

   _____

   _____

   f. Case study: _____

   _____

   _____

   g. Historical research: _____

   _____

   _____

2. Identify a problem amenable to survey research that you would be interested in studying. Outline the kinds of information you would want to collect in the survey. Would you use personal interviews, telephone interviews, or questionnaires to collect your data? Why? Could the same problem be studied using field research methods? Why or why not?

3. Suppose that you were interested in studying a community's need for a food supplement program for low-income pregnant women. How could you use the key informant approach, the survey approach, and the indicator approach to research this problem? Which approach do you think would yield the most meaningful data? Why?

4. Read the article by Parker and colleagues (1993) entitled, "Physical and emotional abuse in pregnancy," which appeared in volume 42 of *Nursing Research* (pp. 173–178). Generate several hypotheses that could be tested by means of a secondary analysis of their data set.

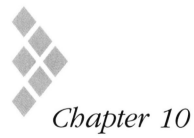

Chapter 10

RESEARCH CONTROL

A. Matching Exercises

Match each "threat" from Set B with a phrase from Set A that indicates the nature of the threat. Indicate the letter corresponding to your response next to each statement in Set B.

SET A
a. Internal validity
b. External validity
c. Neither internal nor external validity

SET B	RESPONSE
1. Selection effects	_____
2. Maturation effects	_____
3. Manipulation	_____
4. Novelty effects	_____
5. Replication	_____
6. Testing	_____
7. Hawthorne effect	_____
8. Experimenter effects	_____
9. Blocking effects	_____
10. Mortality	_____

B. Completion Exercises

Write the words or phrases that correctly complete the sentences below.

1. The environment should be controlled by the researcher insofar as possible by maximizing _____ _____ in the research conditions.

2. The specifications of an experimental treatment are often referred to as the _____ _____ .

3. Randomization serves a general control function in research design by eliminating _____ _____ .

4. Using the principle of homogeneity to control extraneous variables limits the _____ _____ of the findings.

5. When an extraneous variable is dealt with in a randomized block design, the variable is then referred to as a(n) _____ _____ variable.

6. When a repeated measures design is used with more than two conditions, the procedure of _____ _____ should usually be employed to eliminate any ordering effects.

7. When the technique of _____ _____ is used, a subject in one group is paired with a subject in another group with respect to the extraneous variable being controlled.

8. Control over extraneous variables is required for the _____ _____ validity of the study.

9. The differential loss of subjects from comparison groups results in the threat known as _____ _____ .

10. Changes that occur as the result of time passing rather than as a result of the treatment represent the threat of _____ .

11. Events concurrent with the institution of a treatment that can affect the dependent variable constitute the threat of _____ .

12. The group to whom a researcher *ideally* can generalize the research findings is the _____ _____ population.

13. Novelty effects represent a threat to the _____ _____ validity of a study.

14. To help reduce attrition, researchers doing longitudinal research usually collect _____ _____ .

C. Study Questions

1. Define the following terms. Compare your definition with the definition in Chapter 10 of the textbook or in the glossary.

   a. Randomized block design: _____ _____ _____

   b. Matching: _____ _____ _____

   c. Balanced design: _____ _____ _____

   d. Analysis of covariance: _____

_____

_____

   e. Threats to internal validity: _____

_____

_____

   f. Selection threat: _____

_____

_____

   g. External validity: _____

_____

_____

   h. Accessible population: _____

_____

_____

   i. Experimenter effect: _____

_____

_____

2. Examine the 10 research questions in the second matching exercise of Chapter 8. For each, specify one or more extraneous variables that the researcher might want to control.

   1. _____

_____

_____

   2. _____

_____

_____

   3. _____

_____

_____

4. _____
   _____
   _____

5. _____
   _____
   _____

6. _____
   _____
   _____

7. _____
   _____
   _____

8. _____
   _____
   _____

9. _____
   _____
   _____

10. _____
    _____
    _____

3. A nurse researcher is interested in comparing the oral and rectal temperature measurements of febrile adults at two times a day on three different clinical units. Could such a study be conducted as a factorial experiment? Why or why not? If yes, what are the factors in the design? Could this study be conducted as a repeated measures design? Why or why not? If yes, how would you counter-balance? Could a randomized block design be used? Why or why not? If yes, what would the blocking variable be?

4. Below is a list of 10 target populations. For each, think of an accessible population (i.e., a population accessible to *you*) that you might be able to use if you were conducting the study. Be as specific (and realistic) as possible.

a. All pregnant women residing in an urban area _____

_____

_____

b. All high school students applying to schools of nursing _____

_____

_____

c. All parents of children born with spina bifida _____

_____

_____

d. All faculty teaching psychiatric nursing in universities _____

_____

_____

e. All cigarette smokers _____

_____

_____

f. All women using an IUD _____

_____

_____

g. All men older than 45 years of age who have had a cardiovascular accident

_____

_____

h. All licensed midwives _____

_____

_____

i. All male nurses employed in intensive care units _____

_____

_____

j. All patients with hip replacement hospitalized for 7 days or longer _____

_____

_____

5. Suppose you wanted to study the effectiveness of an innovative approach to teaching student nurses how to give subcutaneous injections. In conducting a true experiment for this study, what environmental factors would you want to control with respect to maintaining constancy of conditions?

6. Suppose that you are studying the effects of range-of-motion exercises on radical mastectomy patients. You start your experiment with 50 experimental subjects and 50 control subjects. Your intervention requires the experimental subjects to come for daily sessions over a 2-week period, while control subjects come only once at the end of 2 weeks. Your final group sizes are 40 for the experimental group and 49 for the control group. The results of your study indicate that the experimental group did better in raising the arm of the affected side above head level. What effects, if any, do you think the subject attrition might have on the internal validity of your study?

D. Application Exercises

1. Van Wagner (1995)* investigated the relationship between the use of intrauterine contraceptive devices (IUDs) and the incidence of pelvic inflammatory disease (PID) in a sample of urban women. The data were gathered from the gynecology departments of four health centers (one university, one city hospital, one health maintenance organization, and one consortium of private gynecologists). Van Wagner obtained the records of 600 women—150 from each facility—who were diagnosed within the previous 12 months as having PID. She also obtained the records of 150 women who had come to each of the facilities for some other purpose and who had no record of having had PID within the 12-month period before their focal visit. The two groups of 600 women (the PID and non-PID group) were matched in terms of age (within a 5-year age range of under 20, 20–25, 26–29, 30–35, etc.) and marital status (currently married or not married). For each of the 1200 women, the records were examined to determine whether they had had an IUD inserted within 2 years before their focal visit. For those women for whom no determination could be made based on the records of the facility, brief telephone interviews were administered to obtain the needed information (30 women who could not be reached were replaced with other women to maintain the sample size). The data revealed that 122 women in the PID group (20.3%), compared with 74 women in the non-PID group (12.3%), had used an IUD, a significant group difference. Based on this analysis, Van Wagner concluded that use of an IUD was a cause of PID in this sample.

   Review and critique this study. Suggest alternative designs for examining the research problem. To assist you in your critique, here are some guiding questions:

   *This example is fictitious.

a. Is this research nonexperimental? If so, is it *inherently* nonexperimental? Why or why not?

b. Evaluate the internal validity of the study. What threats to its internal validity, if any, are posed?

c. Examine the criteria for causality presented in Chapter 8 of the text. Does this study meet all the criteria for establishing causality?

d. The researcher concluded that her independent variable (use of the IUD) "caused" a certain outcome (incidence of PID). Can you offer two or more alternative explanations to account for the outcome?

e. What extraneous variables did the researcher identify, and by what method were they controlled? How else might those variables have been controlled?

f. What extraneous variables do you think *should* have been controlled but were not? Why might the researcher have decided *not* to control these variables?

g. To what extent did the researcher control for the constancy of conditions in this study? Suggest ways in which this aspect of the study could have been improved.

h. What is the target population of this study? What is the accessible population? How reasonable is it to generalize the results of this study to the target population?

i. Evaluate the external validity of the study in terms of the "threats" described in Chapter 10. What changes, if any, would you recommend to improve the external validity of the design?

2. Below are several suggested research articles. Read one or more of these articles and respond to questions a through i of Question D.1 in terms of these actual research studies.

- Cole, F. L. (1993). Temporal variation in the effects of iced water on oral temperature. *Research in Nursing and Health, 16,* 107–111.

- Hahn, W. K., Brooks, J. A., & Hartsough, D. M. (1993). Self-disclosure and coping styles in men with cardiovascular reactivity. *Research in Nursing and Health, 16,* 275–282.

- Maloni, J. A., Chance, B., Zhang, C., Cohen, A. W., Betts, D., & Gange, S. J. (1993). Physical and psychosocial side effects of antepartum hospital bed rest. *Nursing Research, 42,* 197–203.

- Tumulty, G., Jernigan, I. E., & Kohut, G. F. (1994). The impact of perceived work environment on job satisfaction of hospital staff. *Applied Nursing Research, 7,* 84–90.

E. Special Projects

1. Suppose that you wanted to compare premature and normal babies in terms of their development at 5 years of age. Describe how you would design such a study, being careful to indicate what extraneous variables you would need to control and how you would control them. Identify the major threats to the internal validity of your design.

2. A nurse researcher is interested in testing the effect of aerobic exercise on the muscle strength and flexibility of sedentary nursing home residents. Describe a design you would recommend for this problem, being careful to indicate what extraneous variables you would need to control and how you would control them. Identify the major threats to the internal validity of your design.

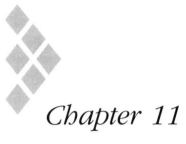

Chapter 11

SAMPLING DESIGNS

A. Matching Exercises

Match each statement relating to sampling from Set B with one of the phrases from Set A. Indicate the letter corresponding to your response next to each of the statements in Set B.

SET A
a. Probability sampling
b. Nonprobability sampling
c. Both probability and nonprobability sampling
d. Neither probability nor nonprobability sampling

SET B   **RESPONSE**

1. Includes systematic sampling   _____
2. Allows an estimation of the magnitude of sampling error   _____
3. Guarantees a representative sample   _____
4. Includes quota sampling   _____
5. Yields better results when the samples are large   _____
6. Elements are selected by nonrandom methods   _____
7. Can be used with entire populations or with selected strata
   from the populations   _____
8. Used to select populations   _____
9. Provides an equal chance of elements being selected   _____
10. Is required when the population is homogeneous   _____

Polit DF, Hungler BP: STUDY GUIDE FOR NURSING RESEARCH:
PRINCIPLES AND METHODS, 5th ed. © 1995 J.B. Lippincott Company.

B. Completion Exercises

Write the words or phrases that correctly complete the sentences below.

1. A(n) _____
   _____ is a subset of the units that comprise the population.

2. The main criterion for evaluating a sample is its _____
   _____ .

3. A sample would be considered _____
   _____ if it systematically overrepresented or un-
   derrepresented a segment of the population.

4. If a population is completely _____
   _____ with respect to key attributes, then any sample
   is as good as any other.

5. Another term used for convenience sample is _____
   _____ .

6. Quota samples are essentially convenience samples from selected _____
   _____ of the
   population.

7. A type of purposive sampling used in in-depth qualitative studies is _____
   _____ sam-
   pling.

8. The most basic type of probability sampling is referred to as _____
   _____ .

9. When disproportionate sampling is used, an adjustment procedure known as
   _____
   _____ is normally used to estimate population values.

10. Another term used to refer to cluster sampling is _____
    _____ sampling.

11. In systematic samples, the distance between selected elements is referred to as the _____
_____ .

12. Differences between population values and sample values are referred to as
_____
_____ .

13. If a researcher has confidence in his or her sampling design, the results of a study can reasonably be generalized to the _____
_____ population.

14. As the size of a sample _____
_____ , the probability of drawing a deviant sample diminishes.

15. If a researcher wanted to draw a systematic sample of 100 from a population of 3000, the sampling interval would be _____
_____ .

C. Study Questions

1. Define the following terms. Compare your definition with the definition in Chapter 11 of the textbook or in the glossary.

   a. Sampling: _____
   _____
   _____

   b. Elements: _____
   _____
   _____

   c. Probability sampling: _____
   _____
   _____

d. Nonprobability sampling: _____

_____

_____

e. Stratum: _____

_____

_____

f. Eligibility criteria: _____

_____

_____

g. Convenience sample: _____

_____

_____

h. Snowball sampling: _____

_____

_____

i. Quota sample: _____

_____

_____

j. Judgmental sampling: _____

_____

_____

k. Random sample: _____

_____

_____

l. Sampling frame: _____

_____

_____

m. Stratified random sampling: _____

_____

_____

n. Disproportionate sampling design: _____

_____

o. Cluster sampling: _____

_____

p. Systematic sampling: _____

_____

q. Screening instrument: _____

_____

2. Using the table of random numbers presented in Table 8-1, select a random sample of 30 names, drawn from a sampling frame of your choice (e.g., a page from a telephone directory, roster of nursing students, a staff list, etc.).

3. For each of the following target populations, identify an accessible population (accessible to *you*) that might be used in a study.

TARGET POPULATION	**ACCESSIBLE POPULATION**
a. All teenagers diagnosed as having scoliosis in the United States	_____
b. All nursing home residents over the age of 70 years in the United States	_____
c. All individuals eligible to receive Medicaid	_____
d. All rape victims in the United States	_____
e. All individuals with blood type O positive	_____

4. Identify the type of sampling design used in the following examples:

a. Thirty inmates randomly sampled from a random selection of five federal penitentiaries _____

_____

_____

b. All the nurses participating in a continuing education seminar _____

_____

_____

c. Every 20th patient admitted to the emergency room between January and
June _____

_____

_____

d. The first 20 male and the first 20 female patients admitted to the hospital with
hypothermia _____

_____

_____

e. A sample of 250 members randomly selected from a roster of American
Nurses' Association members _____

_____

_____

5. Nurse A is planning to study the effects of maternal stress, maternal depression,
maternal age, family economic resources, and social support on a child's socioemotional development among both intact and mother-headed families. Nurse B
is planning to study body position on patients' respiratory functioning. Describe
the kinds of samples that the two nurses would need to use. Which nurse would
need the larger sample? Defend your answer.

D. Application Exercises

1. Krout (1994)* studied the job-search strategies of recent nursing school graduates. Her survey focused on such issues as timing of job applications, number of
applications, source of information about jobs, method of initial contact, and so
on. She was interested in learning whether certain strategies were more successful in achieving job offers (and acceptable job offers) than others. She obtained
lists of graduates from six schools of nursing in Greater Boston (two schools for
each of three different types of programs). She then conducted telephone interviews with 100 graduates from each of the three program types (bachelors,
diploma, and associates). Her method was to find, using local telephone directo-

*This example is fictitious.

ries, the telephone numbers for as many of the names on her lists as she could and to make calls until she had completed 100 interviews with graduates from each group. Thus, her final sample consisted of 300 recently graduated RNs.

Review and critique this research effort. Suggest alternative sampling designs. To assist you in your critique, here are some guiding questions:

a. What type of sampling design was used? Was this design appropriate? Would you recommend a different sampling approach? Why or why not? What are the advantages of the approach used? What are the disadvantages?

b. Identify what you believe to be the target and accessible populations in this study. How representative do you feel the accessible population is of the target population? How representative is the sample of this accessible population? What are some of the possible sources of sampling bias?

c. Did the researcher use a proportionate or disproportionate sampling plan? Is this appropriate? Why or why not?

d. Comment on the size of the sample. Does this sample size appear to be adequate?

2. Below are several suggested research articles. Read the introductory and methods sections of one or more of these articles and respond to questions a through d of Question D.1 in terms of these actual research studies.

- Burgener, S. C., & Shimer, R. (1993). Variables related to caregiver behaviors with cognitively impaired elders in institutional settings. *Research in Nursing and Health, 16,* 193–202.
- Cronin-Stubbs, D., Duchene, P., LeSage, J., Dean-Baar, S., DiFilippo, J. M., Kopanke, D., Stehlin, M., & Swanson, B. (1994). Evaluating a geriatric rehabilitation continuing education program for nursing home and home health agency nurses. *Applied Nursing Research, 7,* 91–93.
- Ganong, L. (1993). Nurses' perceptions of married and unmarried pregnant patients. *Western Journal of Nursing Research, 15,* 352–362.
- Korniewicz, D. M., Kirwin, M., Cresci, K., Markut, C., & Larson, E. (1992). In-use comparison of latex gloves in two high-risk units. *Heart and Lung, 21,* 81–84.
- Staggers, N., & Mills, M. E. (1994). Nurse-computer interaction: Staff performance outcomes. *Nursing Research, 43,* 144–150.

E. Special Projects

1. Suppose that you were interested in studying preventive health care behaviors among low-income urban residents. Describe how you might select a sample for your study using the following:

    a. A convenience sample

    b. A quota sample

    c. A cluster sample

2. Propose a researchable problem statement. Specify a research and sampling design to study this problem. In particular, specify the following:

    a. The target population

    b. An accessible population

    c. Specific eligibility criteria for sampling

    d. A sampling design, together with a rationale

    e. A recommended sample size

With respect to the latter three aspects, be realistic. Take into account your resources, time, and level of expertise. That is, recommend a plan that would be feasible to implement.

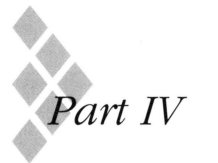

Part IV

MEASUREMENT AND DATA COLLECTION

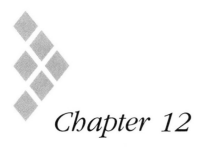

Chapter 12

DESIGNING AND IMPLEMENTING A DATA COLLECTION PLAN

A. Matching Exercises

Match each descriptive statement regarding data collection methods from Set B with one (or more) of the statements from Set A. Indicate the letter(s) corresponding to your response next to each item in Set B.

SET A
a. Self-reports
b. Observations
c. Biophysiologic measures
d. None of the above

SET B   RESPONSE

1. Cannot easily be gathered unobtrusively   _____
2. Can be biased by the subject's desire to "look good"   _____
3. Can be used to gather data from infants   _____
4. Is rarely used in qualitative studies   _____
5. Is a good way to obtain information about human *behavior*   _____
6. Can be biased by the researcher's values and beliefs   _____
7. Can be combined with other data collection methods in a single study   _____
8. Can range from highly unstructured to highly structured data   _____

9. Can yield quantitative information   _____

10. Benefits from pretesting   _____

B. *Completion Exercises*

Write the words or phrases that correctly complete the sentences below.

1. The four dimensions along which data collection methods can vary are _____

   _____ , _____ , _____ , and _____

   _____ .

2. _____

   _____ is especially likely to lead to distortions on the part of subjects who are

   engaged in socially unacceptable behavior.

3. The type of data collection approach that is especially high on objectivity is

   _____

   _____ .

4. When we want to know what people's attitudes are, we are most likely to use the

   method of _____

   _____ .

5. Nonverbal communication would most likely be studied using the method of

   _____

   _____ .

6. In a quantitative study, the first step is usually to create an inventory of _____

   _____ .

7. When a researcher analyzes outcomes for a subset of the sample, this is called a

   search for _____

   _____ .

8. In selecting an existing instrument for use in a study, the primary consideration is

   _____

   _____ .

9. If the population has literacy problems, it may be important to assess a self-report instrument for its _____

_____ .

10. If an instrument is copyrighted, it is necessary to obtain _____

_____ before it can be used.

11. An instrument package should be _____

_____ to determine the amount of time it takes to collect the data.

12. Data collection _____

_____ spell out the specific procedures to be used in collecting the data.

C. Study Questions

1. Define the following terms. Compare your definition with the definition in Chapter 12 of the textbook or in the glossary.

a. Instrument: _____

_____

_____

b. Objectivity: _____

_____

_____

c. Self-report: _____

_____

_____

d. Observer bias: _____

_____

_____

e. Manipulation check: _____

_____

_____

f. Norms: _____

_____

_____

g. Training manual: _____

_____

_____

h. Q-by-Q: _____

_____

_____

2. Below are several research problems. Indicate what methods of data collection (self-report, observation, biophysiologic measures) you might recommend using for each. Defend your response.

a. How does an elderly patient manage the transition from hospital to home?

_____

_____

b. What are the predictors of intravenous site symptoms? _____

_____

_____

c. What are the factors associated with smoking during pregnancy? _____

_____

_____

d. To what extent and in what manner do nurses interact differently with male and female patients? _____

_____

_____

e. What are the coping mechanisms of parents whose infants are long-term patients in neonatal intensive care units? _____

_____

_____

3. For each of the research problems in Question C.2, indicate where on the four dimensions discussed in this chapter (structure, quantifiability, researcher obtrusiveness, and objectivity) the method of data collection would most likely lie.

4. Read the following article and describe the data collection instruments in terms of the four dimensions discussed in this chapter:

   • Pickler, R. H. (1993). Premature infant-nurse caregiver interaction. *Western Journal of Nursing Research, 15,* 548–559.

5. Read one of the following studies, which relied exclusively on self-report, and identify variables that *could* have been measured with an alternative approach:

   • McSweeney, J. C. (1993). Making behavior changes after a myocardial infarction. *Western Journal of Nursing Research, 15,* 441–455.

   • Nyamathi, A., Jacoby, A., Constancia, P., & Ruvevich, S. (1992). Coping and adjustment of spouses of critically ill patients with cardiac disease. *Heart and Lung, 21,* 160–166.

   • Schirm, V., Gray, M., & Peoples, M. (1993). Nursing personnel's perceptions of physical restraints use in long-term care. *Clinical Nursing Research, 2,* 98–110.

D. Application Exercises

1. Caldwell (1995)* was interested in studying a variety of psychological effects (e.g., stress, self-esteem, depression, body image) among women who give birth by cesarean section. She designed a prospective study that allowed her to compare three groups of primiparas: women who gave birth vaginally, those who had a preplanned cesarean section, and those who had an emergency cesarean delivery. According to the research design, data were to be collected in the sixth month of the pregnancy and then again 2 weeks after delivery.

   When Caldwell began to make a list of the variables she wanted to measure, she realized that the data collection would require a considerable amount of time, particularly with respect to the measurement of the dependent variables. Given the likelihood that levels of pain, fatigue, and lack of concentration might be

*This example is fictitious.

expected to be high in the postpartum period, she decided to focus on a single psychological outcome, namely depression.

Caldwell developed three instrument packages: one for administration during the subjects' pregnancies, a second for administration postpartum, and a third consisting of forms for the extraction of information from medical and hospital records. The variables to be measured in each included the following:

(1) *Predelivery self-report.* Demographic information (age, marital status, employment status and occupation, educational background, etc.); pregnancy history; attitudes toward and expectations about cesarean delivery; level of depression

(2) *Postpartum self-report.* Updated background information (e.g., expected date of return to work, if applicable); perception of the birth experience; levels of fatigue and pain; level of depression

(3) *Medical information.* Weight gain during pregnancy; prenatal history (number of prenatal visits, use of vitamins, sonogram history, etc.); method of delivery and reason for cesarean, if applicable; gestational length; infant status (birthweight, length, Apgar score, etc.)

Based on a colleague's recommendation, Caldwell decided to use the Center for Epidemiological Studies Depression (CES-D) Scale as her main dependent variable. She developed all other questions herself. Caldwell pretested the predelivery self-report instruments with 10 pregnant women and the postpartum instruments with 10 women who had recently delivered, 5 of whom had had a cesarean delivery. Caldwell used a nurse assistant to help her collect the data. The assistant had helped her prepare the instruments, so no formal training was thought to be needed.

Review and critique the description of the overall study. Suggest possible alternative ways of collecting the data for the research problem. To assist you in your critique, here are some guiding questions:

a. Most of the data in this study were collected by self-report. Could the data have been collected in another way? *Should* they have been, in your opinion?

b. Comment on the degree of structure of the instruments used. Would you recommend more structured or less structured instruments? Why or why not?

c. Comment on the researcher's overall data collection decisions and approach to developing the instrument package.

d. Were the instruments adequately pretested?

e. Comment on the researcher's method of actually collecting the data, including the use of other personnel.

2. Below are several suggested research articles. Skim one or more of these articles, paying particular attention to the methods used to measure research variables and collect the data. Then respond to questions a through e from Question D.1 in terms of this actual research study, to the extent possible.

- Agho, A. O. (1993). The moderating effects of dispositional affectivity on relationships between job characteristics and nurses' job satisfaction. *Research in Nursing and Health, 16,* 451–458.
- Buchko, B. L., Pugh, L. C., Bishop, B. A., Cochran, J. F., Smith, L. R., & Lerew, D. J. (1994). Comfort measures in breastfeeding, primiparous women. *Journal of Obstetric, Gynecologic, and Neonatal Nursing, 23,* 46–52.
- Collins, C., King, S., & Kokinakis, C. (1994). Community service issues before nursing home placement of persons with dementia. *Western Journal of Nursing Research, 16,* 40–52.
- Farrand, L. L., & Cox, C. L. (1993). Determinants of positive health behavior in middle childhood. *Nursing Research, 42,* 208–213.
- Karp, D. A. (1994). Living with depression: Illness and identity turning points. *Qualitative Health Research, 4,* 6–30.
- Stuifbergen, A. K., & Becker, H. A. (1994). Predictors of health-promoting lifestyles in persons with disabilities. *Research in Nursing and Health, 17,* 3–13.

E. Special Projects

1. Write out Q-by-Qs for the following questions:

    a. Altogether, how many times have you been pregnant, whether you had the baby or not?

    b. Is there a particular clinic, health center, doctor's office, or other place that you usually go to if one of your children is sick or if you need advice about his or her health?

    c. At any time in the past month, have you been a patient in a hospital *overnight?*

    d. Are you now covered by Medicaid—that is, do you have a valid medical card that covers your medical bills?

2. Read one of the studies suggested in Question D.2. Based on this study, write the Background section (Section I.A. in Table 12-1) for a training manual for this study.

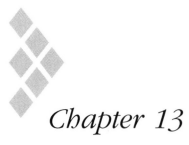

Chapter 13

SELF-REPORTS

A. Matching Exercises

1. Match each descriptive statement regarding self-report methods from Set B with one of the statements from Set A. Indicate the letter corresponding to your response next to each item in Set B.

SET A

a. An interview schedule
b. A questionnaire
c. Both an interview schedule and a questionnaire
d. Neither an interview schedule nor a questionnaire

SET B   RESPONSE

1. Can provide respondents the protection of anonymity   _____
2. Can be used with illiterate respondents   _____
3. Can contain both open- and closed-ended questions   _____
4. Is used in survey research   _____
5. Is the best way to measure human behavior   _____
6. Generally yields high response rates   _____
7. Can control the order in which questions are asked and answered   _____
8. Is generally an inexpensive method of data collection   _____
9. Requires that the purpose of the study be unknown to the
   subject   _____
10. Benefits from pretesting   _____

Polit DF, Hungler BP: STUDY GUIDE FOR NURSING RESEARCH:
PRINCIPLES AND METHODS, 5th ed. © 1995 J.B. Lippincott Company.

2. Match each descriptive statement from Set B with one of the statements from Set A. Indicate the letter corresponding to your response next to each item in Set B.

SET A

a. Likert scales
b. Semantic differential scales
c. Both Likert and semantic differential scales
d. Neither Likert nor semantic differential scales

SET B   **RESPONSE**

  1. Does not permit fine discriminations among respondents   _____

  2. Can be used to measure attitudes   _____

  3. Is sometimes referred to as a summated rating scale   _____

  4. Is subject to response-set biases   _____

  5. Is often used to measure behavioral characteristics   _____

  6. Presents statements to which respondents indicate agree-
     ment or disagreement   _____

  7. Rarely contains more than five items   _____

  8. Uses a graphic rating scale format   _____

  9. Uses item reversals to minimize response-set biases such as
     acquiescence   _____

 10. Provides a quantitative measure of an attribute   _____

B. Completion Exercises

Write the words or phrases that correctly complete the sentences below.

  1. In a focused interview, general question areas are normally listed on a(n) _____

     _____ .

  2. When a group of respondents is assembled in one place to discuss questions
     simultaneously, the approach being used is referred to as a(n) _____

     _____ .

  3. The approach used to question people about important events, decisions, or
     turning points is referred to as the _____

     _____ .

4. A disadvantage of _____

_____ questions is that the researcher may inadvertently omit

some potentially important alternatives.

5. _____

_____ questions are relatively inefficient in terms of the respondents' time.

6. If respondents are not very verbal or articulate, _____

_____ questions are generally

most appropriate.

7. The type of instrument that typically uses more closed-ended than open-ended

questions is the _____

_____ .

8. Questions that offer only two response options are known as _____

_____ items.

9. Another term for two-dimensional checklists is _____

_____ .

10. Likert scales consist of a number of statements written in the _____

_____ form.

11. Some people omit the category labeled _____

_____ in constructing Likert scales, to

avoid "fence-sitting."

12. In Likert scales, positively worded statements are scored in one direction, and the

scoring of negatively worded statements is _____

_____ .

13. Semantic differentials tend to yield measures of three independent dimensions:

_____ , _____ , and _____

_____ .

14. Interviewer probes should always be _____

_____ .

15. Respondents are less likely to give "don't know" responses in a(n) ＿＿＿＿＿

    ＿＿＿＿＿＿＿＿＿＿＿＿＿＿＿＿＿＿＿＿＿＿＿＿＿ situation.

16. Nonresponse in self-report studies is generally not ＿＿＿＿＿＿＿＿＿

    ＿＿＿＿＿＿＿＿＿＿＿＿＿＿＿＿＿＿＿ and can therefore lead

    to bias.

17. The bias introduced when respondents select options at either end of the re-

    sponse continuum is known as ＿＿＿＿＿＿＿＿＿＿＿＿＿＿＿

    ＿＿＿＿＿＿＿＿＿＿＿＿＿＿＿＿＿＿＿＿＿＿＿＿＿＿＿ .

18. Response alternatives should be mutually ＿＿＿＿＿＿＿＿＿＿

    ＿＿＿＿＿＿＿＿＿＿＿＿＿＿＿＿＿＿＿＿＿＿＿＿＿＿＿ .

C. Study Questions

1. Define the following terms. Compare your definition with the definition in Chapter 13 of the textbook or in the glossary.

   a. Unstructured interview: ＿＿＿＿＿＿＿＿＿＿＿＿＿＿＿

   ＿＿＿＿＿＿＿＿＿＿＿＿＿＿＿＿＿＿＿＿＿＿＿＿＿＿＿

   ＿＿＿＿＿＿＿＿＿＿＿＿＿＿＿＿＿＿＿＿＿＿＿＿＿＿＿

   b. Focused interview: ＿＿＿＿＿＿＿＿＿＿＿＿＿＿＿＿＿

   ＿＿＿＿＿＿＿＿＿＿＿＿＿＿＿＿＿＿＿＿＿＿＿＿＿＿＿

   ＿＿＿＿＿＿＿＿＿＿＿＿＿＿＿＿＿＿＿＿＿＿＿＿＿＿＿

   c. Focus group moderator: ＿＿＿＿＿＿＿＿＿＿＿＿＿＿＿

   ＿＿＿＿＿＿＿＿＿＿＿＿＿＿＿＿＿＿＿＿＿＿＿＿＿＿＿

   ＿＿＿＿＿＿＿＿＿＿＿＿＿＿＿＿＿＿＿＿＿＿＿＿＿＿＿

   d. Life history: ＿＿＿＿＿＿＿＿＿＿＿＿＿＿＿＿＿＿＿

   ＿＿＿＿＿＿＿＿＿＿＿＿＿＿＿＿＿＿＿＿＿＿＿＿＿＿＿

   ＿＿＿＿＿＿＿＿＿＿＿＿＿＿＿＿＿＿＿＿＿＿＿＿＿＿＿

e. Interview schedule: _____

_____

_____

f. Questionnaire: _____

_____

_____

g. Open-ended questions: _____

_____

_____

h. Fixed-alternative questions: _____

_____

_____

i. Cover letter: _____

_____

_____

j. Rating question: _____

_____

_____

k. Visual analogue scale: _____

_____

_____

l. Social psychological scale: _____

_____

_____

m. Module: _____

_____

_____

n. Follow-up reminder: _____

_____

_____

o. Probe: _____

_____

_____

p. Response rate: _____

_____

_____

q. Response sets: _____

_____

_____

r. Social desirability response set: _____

_____

_____

s. Acquiescence response set: _____

_____

_____

t. Nay-sayer: _____

_____

_____

2. Below are several research problems. Indicate which type of unstructured approach you might recommend using for each. Defend your response.

a. By what process do parents of a handicapped child learn to cope with their child's problem? _____

_____

_____

b. What are the barriers to preventive health care practices among the urban poor? _____

_____

_____

    c. What stresses does the spouse of a terminally ill patient experience? _____

_____

_____

    d. What type of information does a nurse draw on most heavily in formulating nursing diagnoses? _____

_____

_____

    e. What are the coping mechanisms and perceived barriers to coping among severely disfigured burn patients? _____

_____

_____

3. Suppose you were interested in studying the barriers that low-income women experience in obtaining adequate routine health care for themselves and their children. Develop a topic guide for a focused interview on this topic.

4. For the study described in Question C.3, develop 10 closed-ended questions. Compare the nature of the information you would obtain for the research problem described in Question C.3 using the topic guide versus using the closed-ended questions. Which approach would yield more useful information? Defend your response.

5. Suppose you were interested in studying patients' attitudes toward primary nursing. Develop the following types of questions designed to measure these attitudes.

    a. Dichotomous item: _____

_____

_____

    b. Multiple choice item: _____

_____

_____

    c. Open-ended item: _____

_____

_____

6. Below are hypothetical responses for Respondent Y and Respondent Z to the Likert statements presented in Table 13-3 of the textbook. What would the total

score for both of these respondents be, using the scoring rules described in Chapter 13?

ITEM NO.	RESPONDENT Y	RESPONDENT Z
1	D	SA
2	A	D
3	SA	D
4	?	A
5	D	SA
6	SA	D

Total score:

7. Below are hypothetical responses for Respondents A, B, C, and D to the Likert statements presented in Table 13-3 of the text. Three of these four sets of responses contain some indication of a possible response-set bias. Identify *which* three, and identify the types of bias.

ITEM NO.	RESPONDENT A	RESPONDENT B	RESPONDENT C	RESPONDENT D
1	A	SA	SD	D
2	A	SD	SA	SD
3	SA	D	SA	D
4	A	A	SD	SD
5	?	A	SD	SD
6	A	D	SA	D

Bias:

8. Below are 10 attitudinal statements regarding attitudes toward natural family planning. For each statement, indicate how you think the item would be scored (i.e., would "strongly agree" be assigned a score of 1 or 5, assuming high scores reflect more favorable attitudes?). What are the maximum and minimum scores possible on this scale? Maximum score: _____ ; minimum score: _____ .

STATEMENT	SCORE FOR "STRONGLY AGREE"
a. Natural family planning is an effective method of avoiding unwanted pregnancies.	_____
b. Natural family planning removes the spontaneity from love making.	_____
c. Using natural family planning methods is too time-consuming.	_____
d. A man and a woman can be drawn closer together by collaborating in using natural family planning.	_____

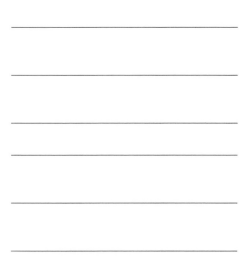

e. Natural family planning is the safest form of birth control

f. Natural family planning is too risky if one really doesn't want a pregnancy.

g. Natural family planning puts a woman in better touch with her body.

h. Natural family planning is an acceptable form of contraception.

i. All in all, natural family planning is the best method of birth control.

j. Natural family planning is "unnatural" in terms of the restrictions it imposes on love making.

9. Identify five constructs of clinical relevance that would be appropriate for measurement using a visual analogue scale (VAS).

10. Suggest response alternatives for the following questions that might appear in a questionnaire.

   a. In a typical month, how frequently do you have sexual intercourse?

   b. When was the last time you had your blood pressure tested?

   c. Which of the following statements best describes your attitude toward nurse practitioners?

   d. What is your marital status?

   e. How would you rate your nursing research instruction in terms of overall quality of teaching?

   f. How often do you skip breakfast?

   g. How important is it to you to avoid a pregnancy at this time?

   h. How many cigarettes do you smoke in a typical day?

   i. From which of the following sources have you learned about the dangers of smoking?

   j. Which of the following statements best describes the physical pain you experienced during labor and delivery?

D. Application Exercises

1. Frantz (1995)* conducted a survey that focused on drug usage patterns in an urban adolescent population. The survey used self-administered questionnaires

*This example is fictitious.

that were distributed to 25 high schools and administered in group (homeroom) sessions to 3568 respondents. The questionnaire consisted of 56 closed-ended and 2 open-ended questions. Included were background questions; questions on the students' attitudes toward, knowledge of, and experience with various drugs; and questions on the students' physical and mental health. The instrument was pretested with 10 college freshmen before administration.

Review and critique the above description of the overall study. Suggest possible alternative ways of collecting the data for the research problem. To assist you in your critique, here are some guiding questions:

a. The data in this study were collected by self-report. Could the data have been collected in another way? *Should* they have been, in your opinion?

b. Were the data collected by questionnaire or interview? Was the decision to use this method appropriate, or would you recommend an alternative procedure? Comment on the advantages and disadvantages of the procedure used for this particular research problem.

c. Comment on the degree of structure of the instrument used. Would you recommend a more structured or a less structured instrument? Why or why not?

d. Was the instrument adequately pretested?

e. Comment on the method in which the instrument was administered. Was the method efficient? Did it yield an adequate response rate? Did it appear costly? What opportunity did respondents have to obtain clarifying information about the questions?

2. Below are several suggested research articles. Skim one or more of these articles, paying particular attention to the methods used to collect the self-report data. Then respond to questions a through e from Question D.1 in terms of this actual research study.

   • DesCamp, K. D., & Thomas, C. C. (1993). Buffering nursing stress through play at work. *Western Journal of Nursing Research, 15,* 619–627.

   • Fawcett, J., Tulman, L., & Spedden, J. P. (1994). Responses to vaginal birth after cesarean section. *Journal of Obstetric, Gynecologic, and Neonatal Nursing, 23,* 253–259.

   • Laryea, M., & Gien, L. (1993). The impact of HIV-positive diagnosis on the individual. *Clinical Nursing Research, 2,* 245–263.

   • McDougall, G. J. (1993). Older adults' metamemory: Coping, depression, and self-efficacy. *Applied Nursing Research, 6,* 28–30.

   • Shaw, C. R., Wilson, S. A., & O'Brien, M. E. (1994). Information needs prior to breast biopsy. *Clinical Nursing Research, 3,* 119–131.

3. Frantz, in her study of drug use patterns among high school students, accompanied each questionnaire with the following cover letter:

Dear Student:

This questionnaire is part of a study to learn about some health-related issues among high school students. Through this study we hope to have a better understanding of young people in America. Students from 25 high schools in the United States are being asked to help us in this effort. Your high school was selected at random.

Your responses to this questionnaire are completely anonymous. No one will know your answers. So, even though some of the questions are very personal, we hope that you will answer honestly. The quality of the picture we will have of high school students today depends on your willingness to provide thorough and honest answers.

Please answer every question. When you are through, please turn the questionnaire in to your homeroom teacher.

Your cooperation in completing this questionnaire is deeply appreciated.

Sincerely,

Carol Frantz, R.N.

Review and critique this sample cover letter. Analyze the tone, wording, and content of the letter. Compare the content with the suggested contents of such a letter presented in Chapter 13 of the textbook.

4. Minnery (1994)† wanted to conduct a survey of nurses' attitudes toward abortion. For this study, she prepared 20 statements pro and con. After developing the items, she asked 10 of her colleagues to indicate their level of agreement or disagreement with the statements, on a seven-point scale. Minnery used the data from these 10 nurses as pretest data for refining the instrument. The original 20 items are presented below:

1. Every woman has a right to obtain an abortion if she does not want a baby.
2. Abortion should be made available to women on demand.
‡3. The government should subsidize the cost of abortions for poor women.
4. Abortions should be made illegal.
5. The right to an abortion should be available to all women.
‡6. Women whose lives are in danger because of their pregnancy should be allowed to have an abortion.
7. Abortion is morally wrong.
8. Women need to have control of their own bodies by having abortion services available to them.
9. Women who have abortions are murderers.
10. People who oppose abortions have no compassion for women's circumstances.
11. Legalizing abortion is a sign of the decay of civilization.
12. No decent woman would even consider killing her own baby through abortion.
13. The freedom to choose an abortion is essential to the liberation of women.
14. An enlightened society gives its citizens the right to make important choices, such as having an abortion.

†This example is fictitious.

15. The right to obtain a legal abortion should never be denied to women.
16. Women who have abortions demonstrate the courage to make a tough decision.
17. No woman should be forced to bear a baby she does not want.
‡18. If men had to bear babies, abortions would never have been illegal.
19. Abortion is one of the most despicable acts that a human can commit.
20. Women should have the right to choose having an abortion.

Upon reviewing the pretest responses, Minnery eliminated items 3, 6, and 18 (indicated with a double dagger). She then had a 17-item scale ready to use in her survey.

Read and critique the description of Minnery's activities. Suggest possible alternative ways of collecting the data for the research problem. To assist you in your critique, here are some guiding questions:

a. What type of scale did the researcher develop? Was this type of scale best suited to the needs of the researcher, or would another type of scale have been more appropriate? Why or why not?
b. Given the aims of the researcher, was the development of *any* type of scale appropriate? That is, could the data have been collected by another method? *Should* they have been, in your opinion?
c. Comment on the procedures used by the researcher to develop the scale. Was the scale adequately reviewed and pretested?
d. Critique the quality of the scale itself. Does it consist of a sufficient number of items? Is the number of response alternatives good? Does the scale do an adequate job of minimizing bias? If not, suggest modifications that might reduce response-set biases.
e. Do you think the scale is unidimensional? That is, does it appear to be measuring one (and only one) underlying concept?
f. Comment on why you think the items that were eliminated (items 3, 6, and 18) were removed from the final scale.
g. Do you feel the researcher needed to develop this scale from scratch?

E. Special Projects

1. Develop a short (2–3 pages) questionnaire, properly formatted and sequenced, for a study of nurses' experiences with victims of child abuse.

2. Draft a cover letter to accompany the instrument developed in Exercise E.1.

3. Develop a topic guide that focuses on nursing students' reasons for selecting nursing as a career and their satisfactions and dissatisfactions with their decision. Administer the topic guide to five first-year nursing students in a face-to-face interview situation. Now administer the topic guide in a focus group setting with

five nursing students. Compare the kinds of information that the two approaches yielded. What, if anything, did you learn in the group setting that did not emerge in the personal interviews (and vice versa)?

4. Develop semantic differential scales to measure attitudes toward the following concepts: cancer, heart attack, AIDS, and brain damage.

5. Describe a potential use for the semantic differential scales described in Exercise E.4. What kinds of comparison might you make in such a study?

6. Construct a VAS to measure fatigue. Administer the VAS two ways: (1) to yourself at 10 different times of the day; and (2) to 10 different people at the same time of day. For the two types of administrations, is there similarity in scores, or is there a wide range of responses? Which of the two yields scores with a wider range?

Chapter 14

OBSERVATIONAL METHODS

A. Matching Exercises

Match each problem statement from Set B with one of the statements from Set A. Indicate the letter corresponding to your response next to each item in Set B.

SET A

a. The study would *require* observational data.
b. The study *could* use observational data as well as other forms of data.
c. The study is not amenable to observational data collection.

SET B   RESPONSE

1. Are nurses' attitudes toward abortion related to their years of
   nursing experience?   _____

2. Are patients' levels of stress related to their willingness to
   disclose their own fears to nursing staff?   _____

3. Are the sleep–wake patterns of infants related to their gestational age at birth?   _____

4. Is the degree of physical activity of a psychiatric patient related to his or her length of hospitalization?   _____

5. Are nurses' scores on a spiritual well-being scale related to
   their degree of comfort in instituting spiritual nursing interventions?   _____

6. Is a child's fear during immunization related to the nurse's
   method of preparing the child for the shot?   _____

7. Does the presence of the father in the delivery room affect the mother's level of pain?   _____

8. Is the ability of dialysis patients to cleanse and dress their shunts related to their self-esteem and locus of control?   _____

9. Is the level of achievement motivation among nursing students related to their clinical speciality?   _____

10. Is aggressive behavior among hospitalized mentally retarded children related to styles of discipline by hospital staff?   _____

B. Completion Exercises

Write the words or phrases that correctly complete the sentences below.

1. The major focus of observation in nursing research is the _____ _____ and _____ of humans.

2. When the unit of observation is small, specific behaviors, the approach is said to be _____ _____ .

3. The reactive measurement effect may occur when the observer is _____ _____ .

4. The technique known as _____ _____ involves the collection of unstructured observational data in which the observer plays a role in the group or culture being observed.

5. The fourth phase of a participant observer's role involves _____ _____ .

6. The three major types of observational positioning in participant observation studies are _____ , _____ , and _____ _____ positioning.

7. The four types of field notes are _____ , _____ , _____ , and _____ notes.

8. In a structured observational setting, the most common procedure is to construct

    a(n) _____

    _____ for observed behaviors.

9. In general, less observer inference is required when the units of behavior being

    observed are _____

    _____ .

10. _____

    _____ is the method of obtaining representative observations without observing all

    behaviors or activities of interest.

11. Observers need to be carefully _____

    _____ in the use of a structured observational

    instrument.

12. One of the major difficulties with observational data is the possibility that the data

    are not _____

    _____ .

13. The tendency for observers to rate things too positively is a bias known as the

    _____

    _____ .

14. An observer bias in which extreme events are given mid-range ratings is known

    as a bias toward _____

    _____ .

15. The tendency for observers to rate things too negatively is a bias known as the

    _____

    _____ .

C. Study Questions

1. Define the following terms. Compare your definition with the definition in Chapter 14 of the textbook or in the glossary.

a. Molar unit of analysis: _____

_____

_____

b. Reactivity: _____

_____

_____

c. Directed setting: _____

_____

_____

d. Log: _____

_____

_____

e. Multiple positioning: _____

_____

_____

f. Mobile positioning: _____

_____

_____

g. Field notes: _____

_____

_____

h. Checklist: _____

_____

_____

i. Sign system: _____

_____

_____

j. Rating scale: _____

_____

_____

k. Time sampling: _____

_____

_____

l. Event sampling: _____

_____

_____

m. Central tendency bias: _____

_____

_____

n. Enhancement of contrast bias: _____

_____

_____

o. Halo effect: _____

_____

_____

2. Below are 10 problem statements in which the dependent variable of interest is amenable to observation. Indicate your recommendation for the relationship between the observer and subjects along the concealment and intervention dimensions for each problem. Justify your response.

   a. What is the effect of touch on the crying behavior of hospitalized children?

   _____

   _____

   b. What is the effect of increased patient/staff ratios in psychiatric hospitals on interpersonal conflict among staff members? _____

   _____

   _____

c. Is the management of appetite loss in burn patients affected by the nutritional information provided by nurses? _____

_____

_____

d. Are the amount and type of information transmitted at the change of shift report affected by the number of years of experience of the nurses? _____

_____

_____

e. Does a patient's need for personal space vary as a function of age? _____

_____

_____

f. Are the self-grooming activities of nursing home patients related to the frequency of visits from friends and relatives? _____

_____

_____

g. Is the adequacy of a student nurse's handwashing related to his or her type of educational preparation? _____

_____

_____

h. What is the process by which very-low-birthweight infants develop the sucking response? _____

_____

_____

i. What type of patient behaviors are most likely to elicit empathic behaviors in nurses? _____

_____

_____

j. Do nurses reinforce passive behaviors among female patients more than among male patients? _____

_____

_____

3. For each of the problem statements indicated above in Exercise C.2, specify whether you think a structured or unstructured approach would be preferable. Justify your response.

a. _____

_____

_____

b. _____

_____

_____

c. _____

_____

_____

d. _____

_____

_____

e. _____

_____

_____

f. _____

_____

_____

g. _____

_____

_____

h. _____

i. _____

j. _____

4. For each of the problem statements listed above in Exercise C.2, indicate whether you think time sampling or event sampling would be preferable. Justify your response.

a. _____

b. _____

c. _____

d. _____

e. _____

f. _____

g. _____

_____

_____

h. _____

_____

_____

i. _____

_____

_____

j. _____

_____

_____

5. Suppose that you were interested in studying verbal interactions among nursing faculty with respect to expressions of solidarity versus antagonism. Would you recommend a molecular unit of analysis (e.g., individual words) or a more molar unit of analysis (e.g., sentences or entire dialogues from staff meetings)? Justify your response.

D. *Application Exercises*

1. Roche (1995)* studied the effect of a school nutritional program on the snacking behaviors of students in grades 1 through 6. During the month of October, the experimental program (which consisted of discussion groups led by the school nurse, posters, and classroom activities initiated by the teachers) was introduced into two elementary schools in a large Eastern city. Two other schools were used as the controls. The children in all four schools were observed with respect to their selection of snack foods, offered once a week at a 2:00-PM snack break. Each snack selected was rated in terms of its nutritional value on a scale from 1 to 9. The observations were made by the school nurses who were in the classrooms and noted the selection of each student. Similar observations were made during the months of October (when the program was implemented) and November (after the program was completed). The data consisted of two main types of information: (1) the frequency with which each snack item was selected each

*This example is fictitious.

week; and (2) the nutritional ratings for the selected snacks for each child. An analysis of these data revealed that the children in the experimental classrooms selected significantly fewer snacks categorized as "nonnutritional salty snacks" (e.g., potato chips) and had a significantly higher average nutritional rating in November than children in the comparison classrooms.

Review and critique this study. Suggest alternative ways of collecting the data for the research problem. To assist you in your critique, here are some guiding questions:

a. The data in this study were collected by observation. Could the data have been collected in another way? *Should* they have been, in your opinion?

b. Specify the relationship between the observer and those being observed on the concealment and intervention dimensions. Do you feel that the specified relationship is appropriate? What kinds of problems might it raise?

c. In terms of the unit of observation, would you describe the approach as basically molar or molecular? Do you think that the level of observation is appropriate, or would you recommend an approach that is more molar or more molecular?

d. Would you classify the study as having used an unstructured or structured observational procedure? Was the amount of structure in the data collection appropriate, or should there have been more or less structure?

e. Was the specific procedure used to measure the study variables an adequate way to operationalize the variables? Could you recommend any improvements?

f. What type of sampling plan was used to sample observations in this study? Would an alternative sampling plan have been better? Why or why not?

g. What types of observational bias do you think might be operational in this study?

h. Comment on the appropriateness of the individuals who made the observations. Can you identify any potential problems with respect to the internal and external validity of the study?

2. Below are several suggested research articles in which an observational approach was used. Review one of the articles and respond to questions a through h from Question D.1, to the extent possible, in terms of this study.

- Brown, S. J. (1992). Tailoring nursing care to the individual client: Empirical challenge of a theoretical concept. *Research in Nursing and Health, 15,* 39–46.

- Davis, T. M. A., Maguire, T. O., Haraphongse, M., & Schaumberger, M. R. (1994). Undergoing cardiac catheterization: The effects of informational preparation and coping style on patient anxiety during the procedure. *Heart and Lung, 23,* 140–150.

- Haber, L. C., & Austin, J. K. (1992). How married couples make decisions. *Western Journal of Nursing Research, 14,* 322–335.
- Helberg, J. L. (1993). Factors influencing home care nursing problems and nursing care. *Research in Nursing and Health, 16,* 363–370.
- McCain, G. C. (1992). Facilitating inactive awake states in preterm infants. *Nursing Research, 41,* 157–160.

E. Special Projects

1. Below is a list of five variables. Indicate briefly how you would operationalize each using structured observational procedures.

   a. Fear in hospitalized children

   b. Pain during childbirth

   c. Dependency in psychiatric patients

   d. Empathy in nursing students

   e. Cooperativeness in chemotherapy patients

2. Develop five problem statements for studies that could be implemented using observational procedures.

3. Develop a problem statement for a study that could be implemented using the participant-observer approach. Analyze the strengths and weaknesses of using this approach for your problem.

4. Suppose you wanted to study facial expressions in autistic children. Describe the sampling plan you would recommend for such a study.

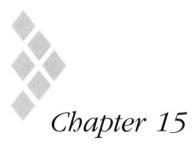

Chapter 15

BIOPHYSIOLOGIC AND OTHER DATA COLLECTION METHODS

A. Matching Exercises

Match each descriptive statement regarding a data collection approach from Set B with one (or more) of the statements from Set A. Indicate the letter(s) corresponding to your response next to each item in Set B.

SET A

a. Biophysiologic measure
b. Vignette
c. Projective technique
d. Q sort
e. Records
f. None of the above

SET B	RESPONSE
1. May be subject to selective survival bias	_____
2. May require advanced training for interpretation	_____
3. Does not depend on respondents' conscious cooperation to provide information about themselves	_____
4. Can measure behaviors and events	_____
5. Is susceptible to response set biases	_____
6. Can be used to measure personality characteristics	_____

Polit DF, Hungler BP: STUDY GUIDE FOR NURSING RESEARCH: PRINCIPLES AND METHODS, 5th ed. © 1995 J.B. Lippincott Company.

7. Can yield or involve qualitative data   _____
8. Is used in most nursing research studies   _____
9. Yields ipsative data   _____
10. Can be administered by mail   _____

B. Completion Exercises

Write the words or phrases that correctly complete the sentences below.

1. Biophysiologic measures that are taken directly within a living organism are

   _____

   _____ measures.

2. The entire set of apparatus and equipment used in connection with biophysio-

   logic measurements is referred to as the _____

   _____ .

3. A(n) _____

   _____ is a device that converts one form of energy into another.

4. The equipment used to amplify or modify an electronic signal is the _____

   _____

   equipment.

5. When biophysiologic materials are extracted from subjects and subjected to anal-

   ysis, the data are referred to as _____

   _____ measures.

6. The major advantage of using existing records is that it is _____

   _____ .

7. In a Q sort, subjects are generally instructed to place most of the cards near the

   _____

   _____ of the distribution.

8. In Q sorts, forcing subjects to place a predetermined number of cards in each pile

   helps eliminate _____

   _____ .

9. Because of its forced-choice nature, the Q-sort technique yields _____

_____

measures.

10. The Thematic Apperception Test (TAT) is an example of the _____

_____ method of pro-

jective techniques.

11. The projective technique in which subjects are presented with a verbal stimulus

to which to react is known as a(n) _____

_____ technique.

12. _____

_____ are brief descriptions of individuals or situations to which subjects are

asked to react.

C. Study Questions

1. Define the following terms. Compare your definition with the definition in Chapter 15 of the textbook or in the glossary.

a. Biophysiologic measure: _____

_____

_____

b. Instrumentation system: _____

_____

_____

c. Records: _____

_____

_____

d. Selective deposit bias: _____

_____

_____

e. Q sort: _____

_____

_____

f. Normative measures: _____

_____

_____

g. Projective techniques: _____

_____

_____

h. Sentence-completion technique: _____

_____

_____

2. Below are five statements that might appear on Q-sort cards. For each, describe different continua according to which the cards could be sorted (e.g., one continuum could be "very much like me/not at all like me" for a statement such as, "I like to go to parties").

a. Americans should change their diets. _____

_____

_____

b. I am bothered by the uncertainty of my prognosis. _____

_____

_____

c. Acid indigestion _____

_____

_____

d. Good fringe benefits _____

_____

_____

e. Freedom from pain _____

_____

_____

3. Indicate which of the measures below is an in vivo measure and which is an in vitro measure:

a. Direct blood pressure measures _____

_____

_____

b. Electrocardiogram measures _____

_____

_____

c. Hemoglobin concentration _____

_____

_____

d. Total lung capacity _____

_____

_____

e. Blood gas analysis of Pco_2 _____

_____

_____

f. Chronoscope measures _____

_____

_____

g. Nasopharyngeal culture _____

_____

_____

h. Goniometer readings _____

_____

_____

i. Palmar Sweat Index _____

_____

_____

j. Blood pH _____

_____

_____

4. Three nurse researchers were collaborating on a study of the effect of preoperative visits to surgical patients by operating room nurses on the stress levels of those patients just before surgery. One researcher wanted to use the patients' self-reports to measure stress; the second suggested using pulse rate and the Palmer Sweat Index; the third recommended using an observational measure of stress. Which measure do you think would be the most appropriate for this research problem? Can you suggest other possible measures of stress that might be even more appropriate? Justify your response.

5. Suppose you were interested in middle-aged people's reactions to the prospect of eventually living in a nursing home. Develop five incomplete sentences that could be used to obtain the information by the sentence-completion technique.

a. _____

_____

_____

b. _____

_____

_____

c. _____

_____

_____

d. _____

_____

_____

e. _____

_____

_____

6. Identify five types of available records readily accessible to nurses that could be used to conduct a research study, and indicate what variables are available from those sources.

a. _____

b. _____

c. _____

d. _____

e. _____

7. What are some of the advantages and disadvantages of a Q sort, as compared with a Likert scale?

ADVANTAGES	**DISADVANTAGES**
_____	_____
_____	_____
_____	_____

8. Below is a study in which vignettes were used. Can you suggest alternative methods of collecting the data? Would the alternative have been preferable in terms of the quality of data obtained?

- Bristow, B, & Nieswiadomy, R. M. (1991). Support of patient autonomy in the do-not-resuscitate decision. *Heart and Lung, 20,* 66–72.

D. Application Exercises

1. Stimmel (1995)* used a combination of projective techniques to study children's fears of hospitalization. Forty children were randomly assigned to an experimental or control condition. The experimental group received a special treatment designed to alleviate prehospitalization anxiety in school-aged children. Controls did not receive any special instruction or treatment. The groups were then compared in terms of their responses to several projective measures, including the following:

*This example is fictitious.

- Responses to three cartoons that showed a hospitalized child interacting with hospital staff in three settings (as the child was being taken to the operating room, as the child was given medication, and as the child was eating). The children were asked to complete the dialogue by indicating the response of the hospitalized child.

- Sentence completions that included the following stems:
  I think nurses are . . .
  Being in a hospital is . . .
  I feel . . .

- Play technique involving the use of dolls. Two dolls are given to the child, and the child is asked to play out a scene between a hospitalized child and a playmate who comes to visit him or her in the hospital.

Read and critique the description of Stimmel's activities. Suggest possible alternative ways of collecting the data for the research problem. To assist you in your critique, here are some guiding questions:

a. Which of the methods described in this chapter did the researcher employ? Was this a good selection? Would you recommend that the researcher switch to an alternative method, such as other methods described in Chapter 15, or in Chapters 13 or 14? Why or why not?

b. Comment on the techniques used in terms of response-set biases.

c. Comment on the techniques used in terms of the degree of objectivity of measuring the critical variables.

d. Comment on the techniques used in terms of the efficiency of the procedure (i.e., amount of time required by subjects and researcher in relationship to the amount of data yielded).

e. Comment on the techniques used in terms of their appropriateness for the study sample.

2. Below are several suggested research articles in which a projective technique was used. Review one of the articles and respond to questions a through e from Question D.1, to the extent possible, in terms of this actual study.

- Logsdon, D. A. (1991). Conceptions of health and health behaviors of preschool children. *Journal of Pediatric Nursing, 6,* 396–406.

- Spitzer, A. (1992). Coping processes of school-age children with hemophilia. *Western Journal of Nursing Research, 14,* 157–168.

- Spitzer, A. (1993). The significance of pain in children's experiences of hemophilia. *Clinical Nursing Research, 2,* 5–18.

- Walker, C. L. (1988). Stress and coping in siblings of childhood cancer patients. *Nursing Research, 37,* 208–212.

3. Wilmot (1994)† conducted a quasi-experimental study of the effectiveness of a program for treating the physiologic anemia associated with pregnancy. The experimental treatment involved instruction regarding a nutritional regimen. The experimental group received verbal instructions by a nurse-midwife regarding dietary requirements and a list of foods known to be high in iron. Recommended daily amounts of certain foods were prescribed. The intervention also involved follow-up telephone conversations with the experimental group members at the 30th and 34th weeks of the pregnancy to discuss dietary and nutritional concerns. The comparison group members were given information that is normally given to pregnant women, with no individual follow-up. Fifty pregnant women who were outpatients at one hospital clinic served as the experimental subjects, and 50 pregnant women who were clients at a health maintenance organization served as the comparison group subjects. Wilmot chose hematocrit readings as the measure of effectiveness of the experimental intervention. During the sixth month of the pregnancy, and again at the 36th-week visit, a hematocrit laboratory test was performed. The data were analyzed by comparing the degree of change that had occurred in the two hematocrit readings within the two groups. The researcher found no significant differences in physiologic anemia in the two groups, as measured by the changes in hematocrit tests.

Review and critique this study. Suggest alternative ways of collecting the data for the research problem. To assist you in your critique, here are some guiding questions:

a. The data in this study were collected by a biophysiologic measure. Could the data have been collected in another way? In your opinion, should they have been?

b. Is the measure used an in vivo or in vitro type of measurement? Is it an invasive or noninvasive type of procedure?

c. Comment on the objectivity of the data collection method. How does its objectivity compare with other methods of measuring the dependent variable (e.g., observations of pallor of the skin, mucous membranes, and fingernail beds)?

d. What other biophysiologic measures might have been used to collect data in the study?

4. Below are several suggested research articles in which a biophysiologic method was used. Review one of the articles, and respond to questions a through d from Question D.3, to the extent possible, in terms of this actual study.

• Bond, E. F., Heitkemper, M. M., & Jarrett, M. (1994). Intestinal transit and body

---

†This example is fictitious.

weight responses to ovarian hormones and dietary fiber in rats. *Nursing Research, 43,* 18–24.

- Lipshitz, M., Marino, B. L., & Sanders, S. T. (1993). Chloral hydrate side effects in young children. *Heart and Lung, 22,* 408–414.

- McCarthy, D. O., Daun, J. M., & Hutson, P. R. (1993). Meperidine attenuates the febrile response to endotoxin and interleukin-1α in rats. *Nursing Research, 42,* 363–367.

- Moody, L. E., Fraser, M., & Yarandi, H. (1993). Effects of guided imagery in patients with chronic bronchitis and emphysema. *Clinical Nursing Research, 2,* 478–486.

- Sparks, K. E., Shaw, D. K., Eddy, D., Hanigosky, P., & Vantrese, J. (1993). Alternatives for cardiac rehabilitation patients unable to return to a hospital-based program. *Heart and Lung, 22,* 298–307.

- Wewers, M. E., Bowen, J. M., Stanislaw, A. E., & Desimone, V. B. (1994). A nurse-delivered smoking cessation intervention among hospitalized postoperative patients—influence of a smoking-related diagnosis. *Heart and Lung, 23,* 151–156.

E. *Special Projects*

1. Develop a hypothesis in which each of the following could be used as measurements of the dependent variable:

   a. ECG readings

   b. Glucose concentration in the blood

   c. Vital capacity

   d. Body temperature

   e. ACTH levels

   f. Microbiologic culture of sputum

   g. Blood volume

   h. Blood pressure

   i. Red blood cell count

   j. Reaction time

2. Suppose that you wanted to evaluate the effect of an experimental nursing intervention on the well-being and comfort of cardiac patients. Indicate several biophysiologic measures you might consider using in such a study. Evaluate each of your suggestions with respect to ease of obtaining the data, relevance, and objectivity.

3. Suppose that you were studying patients' opinions about the elements of care that are important to them during hospitalization. Develop 25 statements that might be used in a Q sort for such a study. One example might be "Receive explanation about what is being done to me and why."

4. Using procedures described in Chapter 15, suggest ways of collecting data on the following: fear of death among the elderly; body image among amputees; reactions to the onset of menarche; anxiety; quality of life; nurses' morale in an emergency room; and dependence among cerebral palsied children.

Chapter 16

ASSESSING DATA QUALITY

A. Matching Exercises

1. Match each statement from Set B with one of the phrases from Set A. Indicate the letter corresponding to your response next to each of the statements in Set B.

SET A
a. Reliability
b. Validity
c. Both reliability and validity
d. Neither reliability nor validity

SET B	RESPONSE
1. Is concerned with the accuracy of measures	_____
2. The measures must be high on this for the results of a study to be valid	_____
3. If a measure possesses this, then it is necessarily valid	_____
4. Can in some cases be estimated by procedures that yield a quantified coefficient	_____
5. Can be enhanced by lengthening (adding subparts to) the measure	_____
6. Is always improved when the measure is made more efficient	_____
7. May in some cases be assessed by scrutinizing the components (subparts) of the measure	_____
8. Is necessarily high when the measure is high on objectivity	_____

9. Represents the proportion of true variability in a measure to total obtained variability   _____

10. Is concerned with whether the researcher has adequately conceptualized the variables under investigation   _____

2. Match each statement from Set B with one of the phrases from Set A. Indicate the letter corresponding to your response next to each of the statements in Set B.

SET A
a. Data triangulation
b. Investigator triangulation
c. Theory triangulation
d. Method triangulation

SET B   **RESPONSE**

1. A researcher studying health beliefs of the rural elderly interviews old people and health care providers in the area   _____

2. A researcher tests narrative data, collected in interviews with people who attempted suicide, against two alternative explanations of stress and coping   _____

3. Two researchers independently interview 10 informants in a study of adjustment to a cancer diagnosis, and debrief with each other to review what they have learned   _____

4. A researcher studying school-based clinics observes interactions in the clinics and also conducts in-depth interviews with students   _____

5. A researcher studying the process of resolving an infertility problem interviews husbands and wives separately   _____

6. Themes emerging in the field notes of an observer on a psychiatric ward are categorized and labeled independently by the researcher and an assistant   _____

B. Completion Exercises

Write the words or phrases that correctly complete the sentences below.

1. People are not measured directly; their _____

_____ are measured.

2. The procedure known as _____ _____ refers to the assignment of numerical information to indicate how much of an attribute is present.

3. In measurement, numbers are assigned according to specified _____ _____ .

4. Obtained scores almost always consist of an error component and a(n) _____ _____ component.

5. From a measurement perspective, response-set biases represent a source of _____ _____ .

6. A reliable measure is one that maximizes the _____ _____ component of observed scores.

7. Test–retest reliability focuses on the _____ _____ of a measure.

8. A(n) _____ _____ is an index of the strength and direction of a relationship between two variables.

9. When the values on one variable tend to be high among individuals who score low on a second variable, the relationship is described as _____ _____ .

10. Another term for internal consistency is _____ _____ .

11. Procedures that examine the proportion of agreements between two independent judges yield estimates of _____ _____ .

12. An instrument that is not reliable cannot be _____ _____ .

13. A measure that looks as though it is measuring what it purports to measure is said to have _____ _____ validity.

14. The type of validity that focuses on the representativeness of the subparts of a measure is _____ _____ validity.

15. The type of validity that deals with the ability of an instrument to distinguish individuals who differ in terms of some future criterion is _____ _____ validity.

16. _____ _____ refers to evidence that different methods of measuring a concept yield comparable results.

17. _____ _____ refers to evidence that a concept being measured is different from other similar concepts.

18. An instrument that makes good use of the time required to obtain measurements is described as _____ _____ .

19. An instrument that can make fine discriminations for different amounts of an attribute is described as high on _____ _____ .

20. The four criteria for establishing the trustworthiness of qualitative data are _____ _____ , _____ , _____ , and _____ _____ .

21. When a qualitative researcher undertakes a(n) _____ _____ in the field, he or she has more opportunity to develop trust with informants and to test for possible misinformation.

22. The use of multiple sources of information in a study as a means of verification is known as _____
_____ .

23. The technique of debriefing with informants to evaluate the credibility of qualitative data is referred to as a(n)_____
_____ .

24. The criterion of _____
_____ refers to the objectivity or neutrality of the data.

25. In qualitative studies, a(n) _____
_____ of data and documents by an independent reviewer can verify the dependability and neutrality of the data and their interpretation.

C. *Study Questions*

1. Define the following terms. Compare your definition with the definition in Chapter 16 of the textbook or in the glossary.

   a. Measurement: _____
   _____
   _____

   b. Isomorphism: _____
   _____
   _____

   c. Obtained score: _____
   _____
   _____

   d. Error of measurement: _____
   _____
   _____

e. Reliability: _____

_____

_____

f. Test–retest reliability: _____

_____

_____

g. Reliability coefficient: _____

_____

_____

h. Internal consistency: _____

_____

_____

i. Spearman-Brown prophecy formula: _____

_____

_____

j. Cronbach's alpha: _____

_____

_____

k. Interrater reliability: _____

_____

_____

l. Validity: _____

_____

_____

m. Content validity: _____

_____

_____

n. Criterion-related validity: _____

_____

_____

o. Construct validity: _____

_____

_____

p. Known-groups technique: _____

_____

_____

q. Multitrait–multimethod matrix: _____

_____

_____

r. Triangulation: _____

_____

_____

s. Audit trail: _____

_____

_____

t. Psychometric assessment: _____

_____

_____

2. Use the Spearman-Brown prophecy formula to compute the following:

a. The full reliability of a 12-item scale whose split-half reliability (i.e., based on six items) is .62.   _____

b. The approximate number of items that would have to be added to increase the reliability of a scale from .70 (for 10 items) to .85.   _____

c. The decrease in reliability for a scale with 30 items and a reliability of .90 if five items were eliminated.   _____

3. The reliability of measures of which of the following attributes would *not* be appropriately assessed using a test–retest procedure with 1 month between administrations. Why?

   a. Attitudes toward abortion: _____

   _____

   _____

   b. Stress: _____

   _____

   _____

   c. Achievement motivation: _____

   _____

   _____

   d. Nursing effectiveness: _____

   _____

   _____

   e. Depression: _____

   _____

   _____

4. Comment on the meaning and implications of the following statement:

   A researcher found that the internal consistency of her 20-item scale measuring attitudes toward nurse-midwives was .74, using the Cronbach alpha formula.

5. In the following situation, what might be some of the sources of measurement error?

   One hundred nurses who worked in a large metropolitan hospital were asked to complete a 10-item Likert scale designed to measure job satisfaction. The questionnaires were distributed by nursing supervisors at the end of shifts. The staff nurses were asked to complete the forms and return them immediately to their supervisors.

6. Identify what is incorrect about the following statements:

   a. "My scale is highly reliable, so it must be valid." _____

   _____

   _____

   b. "My instrument yielded an internal consistency coefficient of .80, so it must be

   stable." _____

   _____

   _____

   c. "The validity coefficient between my scale and a criterion measure was .40;

   therefore, my scale must be of low validity." _____

   _____

   _____

   d. "My scale had a reliability coefficient of .80. Therefore, an obtained score of

   20 is indicative of a true score of 16." _____

   _____

   _____

   e. "The validation study proved that my measure has construct validity." ____

   _____

   _____

   f. "My measure of stress was highly reliable in my study of primiparous women;

   you should use it in your study of stress among emergency room staff." ___

   _____

   _____

   g. "My advisor examined my new measure of dependence in nursing home

   residents and, based on its content, assured me the measure was valid." ___

   _____

   _____

7. What aspects of the multitrait–multimethod matrix that follows identify weaknesses in the measures?

	TRAITS	METHOD 1		METHOD 2	
		A_1	B_1	A_2	B_2
Method 1	A_1	(.40)			
	B_1	.38	(.65)		
Method 2	A_2	.36	.50	(.80)	
	B_2	.19	.48	.25	(.75)

D. Application Exercises

1. Wait (1994)[*] wanted to study paternal bonding and attachment among men who had recently become fathers. Her main objective was to compare paternal attachment among men who had participated with their wives in prenatal classes and were present during childbirth with men who had not. In reviewing prior work in this area, Wait was unable to identify a paternal attachment scale that she found suitable to her needs. Therefore, she developed her own scale to measure paternal attachment. Her scale consisted of 10 statements that respondents were asked to rate as "very much like me," "somewhat like me," or "not at all like me." An example of the statements on the scale is, "The birth of my baby aroused sentiments of immediate affection, closeness, and pride." Total scores were obtained by using procedures analogous to those used for summated rating scales. Wait pretested her scale with 30 men within 48 hours of the delivery of their babies. The internal consistency of the scale was assessed using the split-half technique, which, when corrected using the Spearman-Brown formula, yielded a reliability coefficient of .62. In terms of validating the instrument, Wait used two approaches. First, she invited two colleagues who worked in maternal–child nursing to review the 10 statements and evaluate them in terms of content validity. Second, she asked nurses who worked in the hospital maternity ward to provide ratings, on a 0 to 10 scale, of how attached each new father appeared to be, based on the nurses' observations of the fathers' behavior regarding their babies. The correlations between the fathers' scale scores and the nurses' ratings was .56.

   Review and critique this research effort. Suggest alternative ways of assessing the reliability and validity of the instrument. To assist you in your critique, here are some guiding questions:

   a. What method was used to assess the reliability of the instrument? On what aspect of reliability does this method focus? Is this focus appropriate? Should some alternative method for estimating reliability have been used? Should an *additional* method of estimating reliability have been used?

---

[*]This example is fictitious.

    b. Comment on the adequacy of the instrument's reliability. Should the reliability be better? If so, what might the researcher do to improve the reliability?

    c. What method was used to assess the validity of the instrument? On what aspect of validity does this approach focus? Is this focus appropriate? Should some alternative method for estimating validity have been used? Should an *additional* method of estimating validity have been used?

    d. Comment on the adequacy of the instrument's validity. Should the validity be better? If so, what might the researcher do to improve the validity?

    e. Comment on the efficiency, sensitivity, objectivity, and reactivity of the instrument.

2. Below are several suggested research articles. Read one of these articles, paying special attention to the ways the researcher assessed the adequacy of his or her measuring tool. Evaluate the measurement strategy, using questions a through e from Question D.1 as a guide. (Ignore the more technical aspects of the report, such as those that deal with factor analysis.)

    • Algase, D. L., & Beel-Bates, C. A. (1993). Everyday indicators of impaired cognition: Development of a new screening scale. *Research in Nursing and Health, 16,* 57–66.

    • Kuster, A. E., & Fong, C. M. (1993). Further psychometric evaluation of the Spanish language Health Promoting Lifestyle Profile. *Nursing Research, 42,* 266–269.

    • Lareau, S. C., Carrieri-Kohlman, V., Janson-Bjerklie, S., & Roos, P. J. (1994). Development and testing of the Pulmonary Functional Status and Dyspnea Questionnaire (PFSDQ). *Heart and Lung, 23,* 242–250.

    • Martin, L. L. (1994). Validity and reliability of a quality-of-life instrument: The Chronic Respiratory Disease Questionnaire. *Clinical Nursing Research, 3,* 146–156.

    • Miles, M. S., Funk, S. G., & Carlson, J. (1993). Parental stressor scale: Neonatal intensive care unit. *Nursing Research, 42,* 148–152.

3. Below are several suggested research reports on qualitative studies. Read and critique one of these articles, paying special attention to the ways in which the researcher addressed data quality issues. To assist you in your critique, here are some guiding questions:

    a. Does the report discuss efforts the researcher made to enhance and appraise data quality? Is the documentation regarding efforts to assess data quality sufficiently detailed and clear?

    b. What were those efforts? Was any type of triangulation used? Were there member checks? Was there an external audit of the data?

    c. How adequate were the procedures that were used? What other techniques could have been used profitably to enhance and assess data quality? How much confidence do the researcher's efforts inspire regarding data quality?

   d. Given the procedures that were used to enhance data quality, what can you conclude about the credibility, transferability, dependability, and confirmability of the data?

- Bright, M. A. (1992). Making place: The first birth in an intergenerational family context. *Qualitative Health Research, 2,* 75–98.
- Cohen, M. H. (1993). The unknown and the unknowable managing sustained uncertainty. *Western Journal of Nursing Research, 15,* 77–96.
- Collins, B. A., McCoy, S. A., Sale, S., & Weber, S. E. (1994). Descriptions of comfort by substance-using and nonusing postpartum women. *Journal of Obstetric, Gynecologic, and Neonatal Nursing, 23,* 293–302.
- Stuhlmiller, C. M. (1994). Occupational meanings and coping practices of rescue workers in an earthquake disaster. *Western Journal of Nursing Research, 16,* 301–316.

E. Special Projects

1. Suppose that you were developing an instrument to measure attitudes toward "test-tube" babies. Your measure consists of 15 Likert-type items. Describe what you would do to: (a) estimate the reliability of your scale and (b) assess the validity of your scale.

2. Suggest the type of groups that might be used to validate measures of the following concepts using the known-groups technique:

   a. Self-esteem

   b. Empathy

   c. Capacity for self-care

   d. Emotional dependence

   e. Depression

   f. Hopelessness

   g. Health-promoting practices

   h. Health motivation

   i. Body image

   j. Coping capacity

3. Suppose you were interested in conducting an in-depth study of women who had been raped. Describe ways in which you might achieve: (a) data triangulation, (b) method triangulation, (c) member checks.

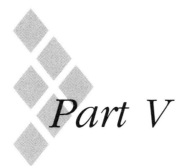

Part V

THE ANALYSIS OF RESEARCH DATA

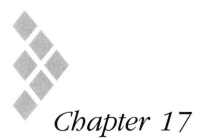

Chapter 17

QUANTITATIVE ANALYSIS: DESCRIPTIVE STATISTICS

A. Matching Exercises

1. Match each variable in Set B with the level of measurement from Set A that captures the highest possible level for that variable. Indicate the letter corresponding to your response next to each variable in Set B.

SET A
a. Nominal scale
b. Ordinal scale
c. Interval scale
d. Ratio scale

SET B	**RESPONSE**
1. Hours spent in labor before childbirth	_____
2. Religious affiliation	_____
3. Reaction time	_____
4. Marital status	_____
5. Temperature on the centigrade scale	_____
6. Nursing specialty area	_____
7. Status on the following scale: nonsmoker; light smoker; heavy smoker	_____
8. Pulse rate	_____
9. Score on a 25-item Likert scale	_____

Polit DF, Hungler BP: STUDY GUIDE FOR NURSING RESEARCH:
PRINCIPLES AND METHODS, 5th ed. © 1995 J.B. Lippincott Company.

10. Highest degree or certification attained   _____

11. Apgar scores   _____

12. Membership in the American Nurses' Association   _____

2. Match each statement or phrase from Set B with one of the phrases from Set A. Indicate the letter corresponding to your response next to each of the statements in Set B.

SET A

a. Measure(s) of central tendency
b. Measure(s) of variability
c. Measure(s) of neither central tendency nor variability
d. Measure(s) of both central tendency and variability

SET B   **RESPONSE**

1. The range   _____

2. In lay terms, an average   _____

3. A percentage   _____

4. A parameter   _____

5. Descriptor(s) of a distribution of scores   _____

6. Descriptor(s) of how heterogeneous a set of values is   _____

7. A standard deviation   _____

8. The mode   _____

9. Can be plotted on histograms   _____

10. Coincide in a normal distribution   _____

B. Completion Exercises

Write the words or phrases that correctly complete the sentences below.

1. Nominal measurement involves a simple _____ _____ of objects according to some criterion.

2. Rank-order questions are an example of _____ _____ measures.

3. With ratio-level measures, there is a real, rational _____ _____ .

4. Unlike ordinal measures, interval measures involve _____

_____ between points on the

scale.

5. A descriptive index (e.g., percentage) from a sample is called a(n) _____

_____ .

6. Researchers using quantitative analysis apply _____

_____ to draw conclusions about a

population based on information from a sample.

7. A(n) _____

_____ is a systematic arrangement of quantitative data from lowest to highest

values.

8. In the equation $\Sigma f = n$, the n represents the total _____

_____ .

9. Histograms and _____

_____ are the two most common ways of presenting frequency

information in graphic form.

10. A distribution is described as _____

_____ if the two halves are mirror images of each

other.

11. A distribution is _____

_____ skewed if its longer tail points to the left.

12. A distribution that has only one peak is said to be _____

_____ .

13. Many human characteristics such as height and intelligence are distributed to

approximate a(n) _____

_____ .

14. Measures that summarize the "typical" value in a distribution are known as mea-

sures of _____

_____ .

15. The symbol $\bar{X}$ is usually used by researchers to designate the _____

_____ .

16. In a positively skewed distribution, the index indicating the "average" value that would be the farthest of the three indexes to the left would be the _____

_____ .

17. Measures of _____

_____ are concerned with how spread out the data are.

18. When scores are not very spread out (dispersed over a wide range of values), the sample is said to be _____

_____ with respect to that variable.

19. The _____

_____ indicates one half of the range of scores within which the middle 50% of the scores lie.

20. The difference between an individual raw score and the mean is known as a(n)

_____

_____ .

21. A squared standard deviation is referred to as a(n) _____

_____ .

22. Statistics for two variables examined simultaneously are called _____

_____ .

23. Another term for a contingency table is a(n) _____

_____ .

24. A graphic representation of a correlation between two variables is referred to as a(n) _____

_____ .

25. Relationships are described as _____

_____ if high values on one variable are associated with low values on a second.

26. The most commonly used correlation index is _____

_____ .

C. Study Questions

1. Define the following terms. Compare your definition with the definition in Chapter 17 of the textbook or in the glossary.

   a. Nominal measurement: _____

   _____

   _____

   b. Ordinal measurement: _____

   _____

   _____

   c. Interval-level measurement: _____

   _____

   _____

   d. Ratio measurement: _____

   _____

   _____

   e. Parameter: _____

   _____

   _____

   f. Histogram: _____

   _____

   _____

   g. Skewed distribution: _____

   _____

   _____

   h. Bimodal distribution: _____

   _____

   _____

   i. Normal distribution: _____

   _____

   _____

j. Mode: _____

_____

_____

k. Median: _____

_____

_____

l. Mean: _____

_____

_____

m. Range: _____

_____

_____

n. Standard deviation: _____

_____

_____

o. Contingency table: _____

_____

_____

p. Correlation matrix: _____

_____

_____

2. For each of the following variables, specify the *highest* possible level of measurement that a researcher could attain.

a. Attitudes toward the mentally handicapped _____

b. Birth order _____

c. Length of labor _____

d. White blood cell count _____

e. Blood type _____

f. Tidal volume _____

g. Scholastic Aptitude Test (SAT) scores _____

    h. Unit assignment for nursing staff _____

    i. Motivation for achievement _____

    j. Amount of sputum _____

3. Prepare a frequency distribution and histogram for the following set of scores, which represent the ages of 30 women receiving estrogen replacement therapy:

```
47  50  51  50  48  51  50  51  49  51
54  49  49  53  51  52  51  52  50  53
49  51  52  51  50  55  48  54  53  52
```

    Describe the resulting distribution in terms of its symmetry and modality.

4. Calculate the mean, median, and mode for the following pulse rates:

```
78  84  69  98  102  72  87  75  79  84  88  84  83  71  73
```

    Mean: _____
    Median: _____
    Mode: _____

5. At the top of page 178 is a contingency table from an SPSS printout. The table presents data from a study of sexually active teenagers in which both males and females were asked how old they were when they first learned about birth control. Each row in the table indicates the ages specified by the respondents. The last row contains the code for respondents who could not remember how old they were, coded 88. Answer the following questions about this contingency table:

    a. How many males were included in the study? _____

    b. How many females learned about birth control at age 14? _____

    c. What percentage of respondents were 16 years of age when they learned about birth control? _____

    d. What percentage of males did not know at what age they learned about birth control? _____

    e. Of those respondents who were 13 years of age when they learned about birth control, what percentage was female? _____

6. Write out the meaning of each of the following symbols:

    a. Σ _____

    b. $\bar{X}$ _____

```
* * * * * * * * * * * * * * * * * * * *C R O S S T A B U L A T I O N
      V276         HOW OLD WHEN FIRST LEARNED BC                    BY SEX
* * * * * * * * * * * * * * * * * * * * * * * * * * * * * * * * * * *

                     SEX
           COUNT   I
           ROW PCT I MALE,      FEMALE          ROW
           COL PCT I                            TOTAL
           TOT PCT I       1. I       2. I
   V276    --------I--------I--------I
           13. I      13  I     10  I      23
               I    56.5  I   43.5  I    25.3
               I    28.3  I   22.2  I
               I    14.3  I   10.9  I
              -I--------I--------I
           14. I      14  I     16  I      30
               I    46.7  I   53.3  I    33.0
               I    30.4  I   35.6  I
               I    15.4  I   17.6  I
              -I--------I--------I
           15. I       7  I     14  I      21
               I    33.3  I   66.7  I    32.1
               I    15.2  I   31.1  I
               I     7.7  I   15.4  I
              -I--------I--------I
           16. I       8  I      2  I      10
               I    80.0  I   20.0  I    11.0
               I    17.4  I    4.4  I
               I     8.8  I    2.2  I
              -I--------I--------I
           17. I       1  I      1  I       2
               I    50.0  I   50.0  I     2.2
               I     2.2  I    2.2  I
               I     1.1  I    1.1  I
              -I--------I--------I
           88. I       3  I      2  I       5
               I    60.0  I   40.0  I     5.5
               I     6.5  I    4.4  I
               I     3.3  I    2.2  I
              -I--------I--------I
           COLUMN      46        45        91
           TOTAL     50.5      49.5     100.0
```

c. f _____

d. n _____

e. X _____

f. x _____

g. SD _____

h. σ^2 _____

7. Suppose a researcher has conducted a study concerning lactose intolerance in children. The data reveal that 22 boys and 16 girls have lactose intolerance, out of a sample of 60 children of each gender. Construct a contingency table and calculate the row, column, and total percentages for each cell in the table. Discuss the meaning of these statistics.

8. A researcher has collected data on pulse rate and scores on a final examination

for 10 students and would like to know if there is a relationship between the two measures. Compute Pearson's *r* for these data:

Pulse rate: 84 72 82 68 96 64 92 88 76 74
Test scores: 92 84 88 72 68 74 72 90 82 86

D. Application Exercises

1. Fox (1994)* hypothesized that sleeping problems in infants were related to various conditions and experiences during childbirth. Fifty infants aged 3 to 6 months were diagnosed as having severe sleep disturbance problems. A group of 50 infants aged 3 to 6 months who had normal sleeping patterns was used as the comparison group. Fox obtained the hospital records for all 100 children. The two groups were compared in terms of the following variables: amount of anesthesia administered during labor and delivery (none, small amount, large amount); length of time in labor (number of hours and minutes); type of delivery (cesarean or vaginal); birthweight (in grams); and Apgar scores at 3 minutes (score from 1 to 10). Fox found that the sleep disturbance group had significantly longer time in labor than the comparison group. The groups were comparable in terms of the other variables.

   Review and critique this research effort. Suggest alternative measurement approaches. To assist you in your critique, here are some guiding questions:

   a. How many variables were measured in this study?

   b. For each variable, identify the level of measurement that was used.

   c. For each variable, indicate whether the measurement could have been made at a higher level of measurement than the level that was used. If yes, specify how you might measure the variable to obtain a higher level measure.

   d. For two of the variables, write out operational definitions that clearly indicate the rules of measurement for those variables.

2. Below are several suggested research articles. Skim one or more of these articles, paying special attention to the ways in which the research variables were operationalized. Evaluate the researcher's measurement strategy, using questions a through d from Question D.1 as a guide.

   • Alexander, D., Gammage, D., Nichols, A., & Gaskins, D. (1992). Analysis of strike-through contamination in saturated sterile dressings. *Clinical Nursing Research, 1,* 28–34.

   • Bowman, J. M. (1994). Perception of surgical pain by nurses and patients. *Clinical Nursing Research, 3,* 69–76.

*This example is fictitious.

- DiIorio, C., Parsons, M., Lehr, S., Adame, D., & Carlone, J. (1993). Factors associated with use of safer sex practices among college freshmen. *Research in Nursing and Health, 16,* 343–350.
- Fuller, B. F., Keefe, M. R., & Curtin, M. (1994). Acoustic analysis of cries from "normal" and "irritable" infants. *Western Journal of Nursing Research, 16,* 243–250.
- Yarcheski, A., & Knapp-Spooner, C. (1994). Stressors associated with coronary bypass surgery. *Clinical Nursing Research, 3,* 57–68.

3. Nolte (1995)† hypothesized that patients with a high degree of physical mobility would perceive themselves as being healthier than patients with less physical mobility. To test this hypothesis, 120 male patients in a Veterans' Administration hospital were asked to rate themselves on a five-point scale regarding their current physical health (1 = very unhealthy and 5 = very healthy) and to predict the number of days that they would be hospitalized. Forty of these patients had been categorized as "of limited mobility," another 40 were classified as "of moderate mobility," and the remaining 40 were described as "of high mobility." Nolte reported a portion of her findings as follows:

   The self-ratings of physical health were fairly normally distributed for the sample as a whole: 42% rated themselves as neither healthy nor unhealthy; 7% and 21% described themselves as "very healthy" or "somewhat healthy," respectively. At the other extreme, 6% said they were "very unhealthy," and 24% said "somewhat unhealthy." The three groups differed in their ratings, however. In the high-mobility group, 45% said they were either "very" or "somewhat healthy," while only 30% of the moderate-mobility and 15% of the low-mobility groups said this. For the entire sample, the mean predicted length of stay was 14.1 days. The median length, however, was only 12.5 days. For the three groups, the means and standard deviations with respect to predicted length of stay in hospital were as follows:

	MEAN	*STANDARD DEVIATION*
High mobility	7.1	3.2
Moderate mobility	11.9	4.5
Low mobility	23.3	7.4

   In this sample of patients, the correlation between predicted length of stay in hospital and the health rating was .56.

   Review and critique this study, particularly with respect to the statistical analysis. To assist you in this critique, here are some guiding questions:

   a. Was the mode of data analysis (i.e., quantitative versus qualitative) appropriate? Why or why not?

†This example is fictitious.

b. Which of the following types of statistical analysis were used in this example?
   Frequency distribution
   Measure of central tendency
   Measure of variability
   Contingency table
   Correlation

c. Comment on the appropriateness of each statistic reported in the example. Is the statistic appropriate given the level of measurement of the variable? Does the statistic throw away information? Is the statistic the most stable statistic possible?

d. Identify two or three statistics that were not reported by the researcher that could have been reported given the data that were collected. Evaluate the extent to which the absence of this information weakened (or streamlined) the report of the results.

e. Discuss the meaning of the means and standard deviations reported in this example.

4. Below are several suggested research articles. Skim one (or more) of these articles, and respond to questions a through e from Question D.3 in terms of the actual research study. (At this point, ignore the references to tests of statistical significance, which are covered in the next chapter.)

- Bauer, B. J., & Kenney, J. W. (1993). Adverse exposures and use of universal precautions among perinatal nurses. *Journal of Obstetric, Gynecologic, and Neonatal Nursing, 22,* 429–435.

- Evans, B. D., & Rogers, A. E. (1994). 24-hour sleep/wake patterns in healthy elderly persons. *Applied Nursing Research, 7,* 75–83.

- Gardner, D. L. (1992). Conflict and retention of new graduate nurses. *Western Journal of Nursing Research, 14,* 76–85.

- Isenor, L., & Penny-MacGillivray, T. (1993). Intravenous meperidine infusion for obstetric analgesia. *Journal of Obstetric, Gynecologic, and Neonatal Nursing, 22,* 349–356.

- Locsin, R. C. (1993). Time experience of selected institutionalized adult clients. *Clinical Nursing Research, 2,* 451–463.

E. Special Projects

1. Fictitious data from 24 nurses for six variables are presented on the facing page. Compute and present 5 to 10 different statistics that you think would best summarize this information.

2. Ask 25 friends, classmates, or colleagues the following four questions:

SUBJECT NO.	SHIFT[a]	ANXIETY SCORES[b]	SUPERVISOR'S PERFORMANCE RATING[c]	NO. OF YEARS OF EXPERIENCE	MARITAL STATUS[d]	JOB SATISFACTION SCORE[e]
1	1	10	4	5	2	4
2	1	13	4	2	2	5
3	1	8	2	1	1	3
4	1	4	7	10	1	3
5	1	6	9	12	1	4
6	1	9	8	7	1	2
7	1	12	6	8	2	4
8	1	5	4	2	1	5
9	2	10	5	4	2	1
10	2	14	6	1	2	4
11	2	8	5	3	1	5
12	2	15	8	2	2	2
13	2	11	8	7	2	3
14	2	14	7	9	1	1
15	2	1	5	3	2	2
16	2	8	8	6	1	3
17	3	3	7	19	2	4
18	3	7	4	7	1	1
19	3	19	5	1	2	2
20	3	5	6	11	1	1
21	3	8	3	2	1	3
22	3	10	4	5	2	2
23	3	13	6	6	2	1
24	3	14	5	3	1	2

[a]1 = day; 2 = evening; 3 = night
[b]Scores are from a low of 0 to a high of 20, 20 = most anxious
[c]Ratings are from 1 = poor to 9 = excellent
[d]1 = married; 2 = not married
[e]Scores are from low of 1 to high of 5; 5 = most satisfied

- How many brothers and sister do you have?
- How many children do you expect to have in total?
- Would you describe your family during your childhood as "close" or "not very close"?
- On your 14th birthday, were you living with both biologic parents, one biologic parent, or neither biologic parent?

When you have gathered your data, calculate and present several statistics that describe the information you obtained.

3. Develop a problem statement (or a hypothesis) for a nursing research study. Prepare operational definitions that specify measurement rules for the variables in your statement. Identify for each variable the level of measurement your definition implies.

Chapter 18

INFERENTIAL STATISTICS

A. Matching Exercises

Match each phrase or statement from Set B with one of the phrases in Set A. Indicate the letter corresponding to your response next to each of the statements in Set B.

SET A
a. Parametric test(s)
b. Nonparametric test(s)
c. Neither parametric nor nonparametric tests
d. Both parametric and nonparametric tests

SET B	**RESPONSE**
1. The signed rank test	_____
2. Paired *t*-test	_____
3. Researcher establishes the risk of Type I errors	_____
4. Used when a score distribution is nonnormal	_____
5. Offers proof that the null hypothesis is either true or false	_____
6. Assumes the dependent variable is measured on an interval or ratio scale	_____
7. Uses sample data to estimate population values	_____
8. Kruskal-Wallis test	_____
9. Computed statistics are compared to tabled values based on theoretical distributions	_____
10. Yields confidence intervals	_____
11. Used most frequently by nurse researchers	_____

12. Used to compare differences for three groups _____
13. ANOVA _____
14. Pearson's *r* _____
15. Chi-square test _____

B. Completion Exercises

Write the words or phrases that correctly complete the sentences below.

1. Sampling distributions of means have a _____

_____ distribution.

2. The standard error of the mean is estimated by dividing the sample standard

deviation by the square root of the _____

_____ .

3. The Greek letter mu (μ) usually symbolizes the _____

_____ .

4. The degree of risk of making a _____

_____ error is controlled by the researcher.

5. Tests that involve the estimation of parameters are referred to as _____

_____ tests.

6. The term *distribution-free statistics* is sometimes applied to _____

_____ tests.

7. The most commonly used _____

_____ are the .05 and .01 levels.

8. Using a .01 rather than a .05 level increases the risk of committing a _____

_____ error.

9. The _____

_____ test is used to compare two groups on the basis of deviations from the

median.

10. The statistic computed in an analysis of variance is the _____

_____ statistic.

11. In an analysis of variance, the term analogous to the *variance* is referred to as the

    _____

    _____ .

12. Multifactor ANOVA permits a test of differential effects of one variable for all

    levels of a second variable, or a test of the _____

    _____ hypothesis.

13. The nonparametric test analogous to ANOVA is called the _____

    _____ test.

14. In chi-square analyses, observed frequencies are compared with _____

    _____ .

15. Spearman's rho is a nonparametric analogue of _____

    _____ .

16. When both the independent and dependent variables are nominal measures, the

    most commonly used test statistic is the _____

    _____ .

17. Kendall's tau is used when both the independent and dependent variables are

    _____

    ____ measures.

18. A(n) _____

    _____ test would be used to compare the heart rates of three groups at two

    points in time.

19. The _____

    _____ is an index describing the magnitude of relationship between two

    dichotomous variables.

20. If a research report stated that a statistical test yielded a $p > .05$, the result would

    generally be considered _____

    _____ .

C. Study Questions

1. Define the following terms. Compare your definition with the definition in Chapter 18 of the textbook or in the glossary.

   a. Sampling error: _____

   _____

   _____

   b. Sampling distribution: _____

   _____

   _____

   c. Standard error of the mean: _____

   _____

   _____

   d. Point estimation: _____

   _____

   _____

   e. Confidence interval: _____

   _____

   _____

   f. Null hypothesis: _____

   _____

   _____

   g. Type I error: _____

   _____

   _____

   h. Type II error: _____

   _____

   _____

   i. Level of significance: _____

_____

_____

   j. Statistical significance: _____

_____

_____

   k. Nonparametric tests: _____

_____

_____

   l. Degrees of freedom: _____

_____

_____

  m. *t*-test: _____

_____

_____

  n. Analysis of variance: _____

_____

_____

  o. Multiple comparison procedures: _____

_____

_____

  p. Repeated measures ANOVA: _____

_____

_____

  q. Chi-square test: _____

_____

_____

2. A nurse researcher measured the amount of time (in minutes) spent in recreation-
al activities by a sample of 200 hospitalized paraplegic patients. She compared

male and female patients, as well as those 50 years of age and younger versus those over 50 years of age. The four group means were as follows:

	MALE	**FEMALE**
≤ 50	98.2 ($N = 50$)	70.1 ($N = 50$)
> 50	50.8 ($N = 50$)	68.3 ($N = 50$)

A two-way ANOVA yielded the following results:

	F	**df**
Gender	3.61	1,196
Age group	5.87	1,196
Gender × Age group	6.96	1,196

Determine the levels of significance of these results, and interpret their meaning.

3. The correlation between the number of days absent per year and annual salary in a sample of 100 employees of an insurance company was found to be −.23. Discuss this result in terms of significance levels and meaning.

4. Indicate which statistical test(s) you would use to analyze data for the following variables:

   a. Variable 1 is psychiatric patients' gender; variable 2 is whether or not the patient has attempted suicide in the past 12 months. _____

   _____

   _____

   b. Variable 1 is the participation versus nonparticipation of patients with a pulmonary embolus in a special treatment group; variable 2 is the pH of the patients' arterial blood gases. _____

   _____

   _____

   c. Variable 1 is serum creatinine concentration levels; variable 2 is daily urine output. _____

   _____

   _____

   d. Variable 1 is patients' marital status (married versus not married); variable 2 is the patients' degrees of self-reported depression (mild versus moderate versus severe). _____

_____

5. Below is a correlation matrix produced by an SPSS run. The variables in this matrix are as follows:

CMATURE = career maturity test scores
EMPKNOW = employment knowledge test scores
BCKNOW = birth control knowledge test scores
V326 = attitudes toward working mothers
FAMSIZE = number of siblings

Answer the following questions with respect to this matrix:

a. How many respondents completed the Career Maturity test?
b. What is the correlation between employment knowledge and birth control knowledge?
c. Is the correlation between family size and career maturity significant at conventional levels?
d. What is the level of significance between employment knowledge and attitudes toward working mothers?
e. With which variable(s) is career maturity significantly related at conventional levels?
f. Explain what is meant by the correlation between CMATURE and BCKNOW.

```
SPSS BATCH SYSTEM                                         FRI, NOV 20, 1990,  8:48 AM

FILE    NONAME    (CREATION DATE = 11/20/90)
SUBFILE    REDIR1

- - - - - - - - - - -P E A R S O N   C O R R E L A T I O N   C O E F F I C I E N T S - - - - -


             CMATURE    EMPKNOW    BCKNOW     V326       FAMSIZE

CMATURE      1.0000      .4618      .3309      .0057     -.0136
             ( 334)     ( 330)     ( 333)     ( 175)     ( 324)
             S=#####    S= .000    S= .000    S= .470    S= .404

EMPKNOW       .4618     1.0000      .2725      .1502     -.0639
             ( 330)     ( 333)     ( 332)     ( 174)     ( 323)
             S= .000    S=#####    S= .000    S= .024    S= .126

BCKNOW        .3309      .2725     1.0000     -.0129     -.0830
             ( 333)     ( 332)     ( 338)     ( 177)     ( 328)
             S= .000    S= .000    S=#####    S= .432    S= .067

V326          .0057      .1502     -.0129     1.0000     -.0947
             ( 175)     ( 174)     ( 177)     ( 178)     ( 175)
             S= .470    S= .024    S= .432    S=#####    S= .106

FAMSIZE      -.0136     -.0639     -.0830     -.0947     1.0000
             ( 324)     ( 323)     ( 328)     ( 175)     ( 329)
             S= .404    S= .126    S= .067    S= .106    S=#####

(COEFFICIENT/(CASES)/SIGNIFICANCE) (A VALUE OF 99.0000 IS PRINTED IF A COEFFICIENT CANNOT BE COMPUTED)
```

D. Application Exercises

1. Wells (1995)* investigated whether taste acuity declines with age, using a cross-sectional design. Eighty subjects were given a taste acuity test in which they were asked to indicate, for 25 substances, whether the taste was salty, sweet, bitter, or sour. The substances were presented in randomized order. Each person had five scores: four scores corresponding to the correct identification of the substances in the four taste categories, and one total score. Twenty subjects from each of the following age groups were tested: 31–40; 41–50; 51–60; and 61–70. It was hypothesized that taste acuity would decline with age, both overall and for all four subcategories of taste. The mean test scores for the four groups on all five outcome measures are presented below, together with information on the statistical tests performed.

	AGE GROUP (years)				F	df	p
	31–40	41–50	51–60	61–70			
Salty test	6.3	5.8	5.7	5.4	3.5	3,76	<.05
Sweet test	5.0	5.0	5.4	5.2	1.2	3,76	>.05
Bitter test	4.0	4.1	3.7	3.3	2.6	3,76	<.05
Sour test	1.9	2.0	2.0	2.1	0.8	3,76	>.05
Overall test	17.2	16.9	16.8	16.0	2.4	3,76	<.05

*This example is ficticious.

Wells concluded that her hypothesis was only partially supported by the data.

Review and critique the above study. Suggest possible alternatives for handling the analysis of the data. To assist you in your critique, here are some guiding questions:

a. For each of the variables, indicate the actual level of measurement as used; now indicate the highest possible level of measurement for each. Is there a discrepancy? If so, can you think of a justification for it?
b. What statistical test was used to analyze the data? Did the researcher use the appropriate statistical test? If not, what statistical test do you think would be more suitable?
c. Are the degrees of freedom as presented correct?
d. The test statistics shown are associated with a specified p level. Using the tables in the Appendix of the textbook, determine whether these p levels are correct.

*This example is fictitious

e. Which of the results is statistically significant? Describe the meaning of each of the statistical tests.

2. Below are several suggested research articles. Skim one (or more) of these articles and respond to questions a through e from Question D.1 in terms of the actual research study.

- Bruce, S. L., & Grove, S. K. (1994). The effect of a coronary artery risk evaluation program on serum lipid values and cardiovascular risk levels. *Applied Nursing Research, 7,* 67–74.
- Erickson, R. S., & Yount, S. T. (1991). Effect of aluminized covers on body temperature in patients having abdominal surgery. *Heart and Lung, 20,* 255–264.
- Gulick, E. E. (1994). Social support among persons with multiple sclerosis. *Research in Nursing and Health, 17,* 195–206.
- Kearney, M. H., & Cronenwett, L. (1991). Breastfeeding and employment. *Journal of Obstetric, Gynecologic, and Neonatal Nursing, 20,* 471–480.
- Williams, M. A., Oberst, M. T., & Bjorklund, B. C. (1994). Early outcomes after hip fracture among women discharged home and to nursing homes. *Research in Nursing and Health, 17,* 175–183.

E. Special Projects

1. Below is a list of variables. Assume that you have data from 500 nurses on these variables. Develop two or three hypotheses regarding the relationships among these variables, and indicate what statistical tests you would use to test your hypotheses.

- Number of years of nursing experience
- Type of employment setting (hospital, nursing school, public school system, industry)
- Salary
- Marital status
- Job satisfaction ("dissatisfied," "neither dissatisfied nor satisfied," or "satisfied")
- Number of children under 18 years of age
- Gender
- Type of nursing preparation (diploma, Associate's, Bachelor's)

2. Using the data presented in Question E.1 of Chapter 17, perform at least two inferential statistical tests. Write a one-paragraph description of the results.

Chapter 19

ADVANCED STATISTICAL PROCEDURES

A. Matching Exercises

Match each phrase from Set B with one (or more) of the statistical analyses presented in Set A. Indicate the letter(s) corresponding to your response next to each of the statements in Set B.

SET A

a. Multiple regression analysis
b. Discriminant function analysis
c. Factor analysis
d. Canonical correlation
e. Multivariate ANOVA

SET B	RESPONSE
1. Always has more than one independent variable	_____
2. Is based on least-squares principles	_____
3. Yields an R^2 statistic	_____
4. Used to reduce variables to a smaller number of dimensions	_____
5. Has more than one dependent variable	_____
6. Yields a Wilks' lambda statistic	_____
7. Is a multivariate statistical procedure	_____
8. May use a procedure known as principal components	_____

Polit DF, Hungler BP: STUDY GUIDE FOR NURSING RESEARCH: PRINCIPLES AND METHODS, 5th ed. © 1995 J.B. Lippincott Company.

9. Involves a dependent variable that is categorical (nominal level) _____

10. Can involve as few as three variables _____

B. Completion Exercises

Write the words or phrases that correctly complete the sentences below.

1. In the basic linear regression equation (Y = a + bX), b is referred to as the _____, and a is the _____ _____.

2. In a regression context, the error terms are referred to as _____ _____.

3. The square of _____ _____ indicates the proportion of variance accounted for by two or more correlated variables.

4. The _____ _____ coefficient is never less than the highest bivariate correlation between the independent or dependent variables.

5. Independent variables are introduced one at a time in _____ _____ multiple regression.

6. Scores that have been adjusted to have a mean of zero and a standard deviation of one are called _____ _____.

7. Standardized regression coefficients are referred to as _____ _____.

8. ANCOVA is shorthand for _____ _____.

9. In ANCOVA, the extraneous variable being controlled is referred to as the _____ _____.

10. _____

_____ is the procedure that yields mean scores adjusted for covariates.

11. In factor analysis, the underlying dimensions are referred to as _____

_____.

12. The first phase in factor analysis is the _____

_____ phase.

13. In factor analysis, _____

_____ are values equal to the sum of the squared weights for

each factor.

14. The second phase of factor analysis is the _____

_____ phase.

15. In _____ rotation, factors are kept at right

angles to one another, while in _____ rota-

tion, the factors are allowed to be correlated.

16. The procedure known as _____

_____ can be used for classification purposes.

17. The most general multivariate procedure is _____

_____.

18. MANOVA is the acronym for _____

_____.

19. In path analysis, the conceptual causal model is depicted in a _____

_____.

20. A variable whose determinants lie outside of a model in path analysis is called

_____

_____.

21. When a causal flow is unidirectional, the model is said to be _____

_____.

22. In power analysis, the four major factors needed to arrive at a solution are the

significance criterion, the power criterion, the sample size, and the _____

_____.

23. An alternative estimation procedure to ordinary least squares is the _____

    _____

    procedure.

24. When the dependent variable is a measure of the duration of some event or

    characteristic, an analytic procedure that can be used is _____

    _____ analysis.

25. The acronym for the technique referred to as linear structural relation analysis is

    _____

    _____ .

C. Study Questions

1. Define the following terms. Compare your definition with the definition in Chapter 19 of the textbook or in the glossary.

    a. Multivariate statistics: _____

    _____

    _____

    b. Multiple regression analysis: _____

    _____

    _____

    c. Least-squares principle: _____

    _____

    _____

    d. Coefficient of determination: _____

    _____

    _____

    e. Analysis of covariance: _____

    _____

    _____

f. Factor analysis: _____

_____

_____

g. Factor loadings: _____

_____

_____

h. Factor scores: _____

_____

_____

i. Discriminant function analysis: _____

_____

_____

j. Canonical correlation: _____

_____

_____

k. Multivariate analysis of variance: _____

_____

_____

l. Path analysis: _____

_____

_____

m. Mediating variable: _____

_____

_____

n. Power analysis: _____

_____

_____

o. Eta-squared: _____

_____

_____

p. Life table analysis: _____

_____

_____

q. LISREL: _____

_____

_____

2. Examine the correlation matrix below and explain the various entries. Explain why the *multiple* correlation coefficient between variables B through E and Satisfaction With Parenthood is .54. Could it be smaller? How could it be made larger? What is the R^2 for the correlation between Satisfaction With Parenthood and the other variables? What does this mean?

	VAR. A	*VAR. B*	*VAR. C*	*VAR. D*	*VAR. E*
	Satisfaction With Parenthood	*Number of Children*	*Marital Status (Married vs. Divorced/Widowed)*	*Family Income*	*Religion (Catholic vs. Non-Catholic)*
Var. A	1.00				
Var. B	−.26	1.00			
Var. C	.48	.29	1.00		
Var. D	.19	−.22	.68	1.00	
Var. E	.10	.37	.17	−.04	1.00

3. Suggest possible covariates that could be used in the following analyses:

a. An analysis of the effect of family stress on the incidence of child abuse: _

_____

_____

b. An analysis of the effect of age on patients' acceptance of pastoral counseling:

_____

_____

_____

c. An analysis of the effect of therapeutic touch on patients' perceptions of well-being: ───────────────────────────────

──

──

d. An analysis of the effect of need for achievement on students' attrition from a nursing program: ───────────────────────────

──

──

e. An analysis of the effect of faculty rank on faculty members' satisfaction with communication among colleagues: ─────────────────

──

──

4. In the following examples, which multivariate procedure is most appropriate for analyzing the data?

a. A researcher is testing the effect of verbal expressiveness, self-esteem, age, and the availability of family supports among a group of recently discharged psychiatric patients on recidivism (i.e., whether they will be readmitted within 12 months after discharge). ──────────────────────

──

b. A researcher is comparing the bereavement and coping processes of recently widowed versus divorced individuals, controlling for their age and length of marriage. ────────────────────────────────────

──

c. A researcher wants to test the effects of (a) two drug treatments and (b) two dosages of each drug on (a) blood pressure and (b) the pH and Po_2 levels of arterial blood gases. ──────────────────────────────

──

d. A researcher wants to predict hospital staff absentee rates based on month of the year, staff rank, shift, number of years with the hospital, and marital status.

_____

_____

5. Below is a list of variables that a nurse researcher might be interested in predicting. For each, suggest at least three independent variables that could be used in a multiple regression analysis.

a. Leadership in nursing supervisors: _____

_____

_____

b. Nurses' frequency of administering pain medication: _____

_____

_____

c. Proficiency in doing patient interviews: _____

_____

_____

d. Patient satisfaction with nursing care: _____

_____

_____

e. Anxiety levels of prostatectomy patients: _____

_____

_____

6. Flett, Harcourt, and Alpass, in their 1994 study of the psychosocial aspects of chronic lower leg ulceration in the elderly (*Western Journal of Nursing Research, 16,* 183–192), used a series of *t*-tests to compare various psychosocial attributes in older people with and without chronic lower leg ulceration. Identify two or three multivariate procedures that could have been used to analyze the data, being as specific as possible (e.g., if you suggest ANCOVA, identify appropriate covariates).

D. *Application Exercises*

1. Milot (1995)* studied psychological distress and life satisfaction in a sample of 100 infertile couples. She hypothesized that the individuals' psychological reactions would differ depending on whether the fertility problem was their own or that of their partners. She further hypothesized that women would be more negatively affected psychologically than men by the fertility problem. Milot administered anonymous questionnaires to both husbands and wives who were patients at an infertility clinic. In 50 couples, the fertility problem was diagnosed as a male problem, and in the remaining 50 couples, it was diagnosed as a female problem. The questionnaire included a set of 50 items, designed to measure psychological well-being. The items included such statements as, "I have felt moments of severe depression lately" and, "My husband (wife) and I have been less communicative than usual." Respondents were asked to indicate whether each statement was "very much like me," "somewhat like me," or "not at all like me." Responses to the 50 items were then factor analyzed. Four factors were extracted and rotated orthogonally. Milot labeled the four factors as follows: "depression," "marital satisfaction," "optimism about the future," and "feelings of gender-role inadequacies." The factor scores on these four scales were analyzed in four separate (2 × 2) analyses of covariance, using the women's age and duration of the marriage as covariates. The following table summarizes the results of the statistical tests for the main and interaction effects (for each test there are 1 and 194 degrees of freedom):

	GENDER OF PARTNER (Male versus female)	*LOCUS OF FERTILITY PROBLEMS* (Self versus partner)	*GENDER × LOCUS INTERACTION*
Depression	$F = 5.9$*; $p < .05$	$F = 6.7$†; $p < .01$	$F = 3.9$; $p < .05$
Marital satisfaction	$F = 0.8$ ns	$F = 1.4$; $p < .05$	$F = 2.3$ ns
Optimism	$F = 1.9$ ns	$F = 2.1$ ns	$F = 1.5$ ns
Gender-role inadequacy	$F = 5.2$*; $p < .05$	$F = 11.4$†; $p < .001$	$F = 3.1$ ns

*Wife higher than husband
†Self higher than partner
ns, Not statistically significant.

Milot concluded that her hypotheses were partially supported by the data.

Review and critique this study with respect to the analysis of the data. To assist you in your critique, here are some guiding questions:

*This example is fictitious.

a. For each variable in the study, what is the level of measurement?

b. How many independent and dependent variables are there in this study?

c. Considering responses to the above two questions and the size of the sample, did the researcher use the appropriate analysis? Suggest alternative ways to analyze the data and compare the information yielded in the two approaches.

d. The test statistics shown are associated with a specific *p* level. Using the tables in the Appendix of the text, determine whether each *p* level is correct.

e. What does each of the statistical tests signify?

2. Below are several suggested research articles. Read one of these articles, paying special attention to the analysis of the data. Respond to questions a through e from Question D.1. in terms of the actual research study.

- Cossette, S., & Levesque, L. (1993). Caregiving tasks as predictors of mental health of wife caregivers of men with chronic obstructive pulmonary disease. *Research in Nursing and Health, 16,* 251–263.

- Duckett, L., Henly, S. J., & Garvis, M. (1993). Predicting breastfeeding duration during the postpartum hospitalization. *Western Journal of Nursing Research, 15,* 177–193.

- Gilliss, C. L., Gortner, S. R., Hauck, W. W., Shinn, J. A., Sparacino, P. A., & Tompkins, C. (1993). A randomized clinical trial of nursing care for recovery from cardiac surgery. *Heart and Lung, 22,* 125–133.

- Melnyk, B. M. (1994). Coping with unplanned childhood hospitalization: Effects of informational interventions on mothers and children. *Nursing Research, 43,* 50–55.

- Metheny, N., Reed, L., Wiersema, L., McSweeney, M., Wehrle, M. A., & Clark, J. (1993). Effectiveness of pH measurements in predicting feeding tube placement: An update. *Nursing Research, 42,* 324–331.

- Rizzuto, C., Bostruom, J., Suter, W. N., & Chenitz, W. C. (1994). Predictors of nurses' involvement in research activities. *Western Journal of Nursing Research, 16,* 193–204.

E. *Special Projects*

1. On the following page is a rotated factor matrix for a set of 20 Likert items administered to 300 teenagers in a study of teenaged sexuality and contraceptive practices.

Using this matrix, do the following:

a. Identify and label the underlying dimensions.

b. Select the items that will form three scales.

c. Compute factor scores for three individuals whose responses to the 20 items are as follows:

Mary:	1	2	5	3	5	4	2	3	4	4	3	1	1	4	2	1	4	1	2	4
Tom:	4	1	2	4	1	2	5	4	1	3	1	2	4	2	1	3	4	5	2	3
Debbie:	2	4	1	2	2	1	5	1	2	4	4	5	2	2	5	1	1	4	5	4

2. Design and describe a study in which you would use both factor analysis and discriminant function analysis.

3. Design and describe a study in which you would use life table analysis.

ITEM	*FACTOR I*	*FACTOR II*	*FACTOR III*
1. It is primarily the woman's responsibility to use birth control.	.10	.62	.22
2. It is difficult to talk to your boyfriend about what kind of birth control the two of you should use.	.09	−.07	.36
3. It can be exciting to take a chance on getting pregnant.	.72	−.03	.08
4. It is relatively easy to put the worry about pregnancy out of one's mind.	.18	−.02	.25
5. It is sometimes important to prove your love by taking a chance.	.48	−.21	.13
6. No form of birth control really works.	.18	.06	−.18
7. People are foolish to depend on luck when it comes to pregnancy risk.	−.40	.17	−.23
8. Every teen who really wants to use birth control can easily do so.	.16	−.02	−.47
9. Sometimes making love with a particular person is worth the chance of pregnancy.	.51	.11	−.12
10. The best birth control methods are those that the man uses.	−.09	−.42	.17
11. A woman sometimes has a really hard time avoiding sexual involvement even when there isn't any birth control available.	.05	−.04	.32
12. The problem with some birth control is that you have to plan for the possibility of intercourse ahead of time.	−.04	.03	.52
13. A woman can't really trust a man to handle contraception.	−.01	.39	.07
14. If you really love someone, the chances of pregnancy aren't so important.	.36	.12	−.01
15. Getting hold of good birth control is a lot of effort and bother.	.02	−.09	.61

(continued)

(continued)

ITEM	FACTOR I	FACTOR II	FACTOR III
16. A woman needs to be in control of birth control for her own protection.	.03	.43	−.15
17. It's pretty easy to protect oneself against a pregnancy.	−.11	.06	−.68
18. Having unprotected sex isn't worth the risk of disrupting your life.	−.58	−.07	.24
19. It's really a hassle to use birth control.	.22	−.01	.49
20. It's a man's duty to see that his partner is protected.	.08	−.47	−.20

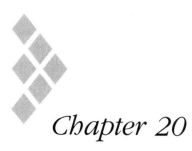

Chapter 20

COMPUTERS AND
SCIENTIFIC RESEARCH

A. Matching Exercises

1. Match each statement from Set B with one of the terms in Set A. Indicate the letter corresponding to your response next to each of the statements in Set B.

SET A
a. Computer hardware
b. Computer software
c. Neither hardware nor software
d. Both hardware and software

SET B	**RESPONSE**
1. Includes the central processing unit	_____
2. Facilitates the analysis of research data	_____
3. Is read into the computer by input devices	_____
4. Makes use of programming languages	_____
5. Is the part of the computer that does the thinking	_____
6. Includes magnetic disk drives	_____
7. SPSS is one example	_____
8. Requires electronics expertise to design	_____
9. Includes the data collected by a researcher	_____
10. Can be networked	_____

Polit DF, Hungler BP: STUDY GUIDE FOR NURSING RESEARCH: PRINCIPLES AND METHODS, 5th ed. © 1995 J.B. Lippincott Company.

2. Match each variable listed in Set B with a field-width specification listed in Set A. Indicate the letter corresponding to your response (i.e., for the maximum field-width needed) next to each of the statements in Set B.

SET A

a. One-digit field-width
b. Two-digit field-width
c. Three-digit field-width
d. Four-digit field-width
e. Five-digit field-width or wider

SET B   **RESPONSE**

 1. Infant's birthweight (in ounces)   _____

 2. Nurse's annual salary (in dollars)   _____

 3. Number of beds in Hospital X   _____

 4. Response to a Likert-type item   _____

 5. Pulse rate   _____

 6. Marital status   _____

 7. Number of hours in surgery   _____

 8. Tidal volume   _____

 9. Weekly aspirin consumption   _____

10. Height in inches   _____

11. Number of cigarettes smoked per week   _____

12. Number of pregnancies   _____

13. Systolic blood pressure   _____

14. Student enrollment in a school of nursing   _____

15. Religion   _____

B. Completion Exercises

Write the words or phrases that correctly complete the sentences below.

 1. The most distinctive characteristic of computers is their _____

   _____ .

 2. _____

   _____ are the things that computers can be used to do.

3. Microcomputers are more commonly known as _____

_____ .

4. I/O stands for _____

_____ .

5. Data are read in through some form of _____

_____ .

6. CPU stands for _____

_____ .

7. The computer _____

_____ is composed of a series of cells, each of which stores an

instruction or numerical value.

8. A megabyte is equal to _____

_____ bytes.

9. A set of instructions to the computer is referred to as a(n) _____

_____ .

10. FORTRAN and BASIC are examples of _____

_____ .

11. Word processing and spreadsheets are examples of _____

_____ .

12. The main difference between IBM-compatible computers and Macs is their

_____

_____ .

13. Two main input devices for a personal computer are the _____

_____ and _____ .

14. Disks can be used as input and output devices and also as _____

_____ storage devices.

15. MD-DOS and OS/2 are both examples of _____

_____ for IBM-type computers.

16. The instructions that help the computer "pull itself up" are known as the _____

_____ .

17. For security reasons, legitimate users of computer facilities often need a(n) _____ and a(n) _____ _____ .

18. The acronym LAN stands for _____ _____ .

19. To access an electronic bulletin board, the hardware of your computer would need to include a(n) _____ _____ .

20. SPSS, SAS, and BMD-P are examples of _____ _____ .

21. Coding of research data for statistical analysis should ideally involve _____ _____ symbols.

22. Variables measured on the _____ _____ scale can be assigned an arbitrary code.

23. Variables that are inherently _____ _____ do not need to be coded.

24. Closed-ended questions can usually be _____ _____ .

25. In coding open-ended or unstructured materials, the coding categories should be mutually exclusive and _____ _____ .

26. "Don't knows" and refusals must be treated as _____ _____ .

27. Each individual case (e.g., each respondent) in a study should be assigned a unique _____ _____ .

28. _____ _____ procedures are recommended to detect errors in data entry.

29. Entered data are not ready for analysis until they have been _____ _____ .

30. Coding and data entry decisions should be fully _____

_____ .

C. *Study Questions*

1. Define the following terms. Compare your definition with the definition in Chapter 20 of the textbook or in the glossary.

   a. Computer hardware: _____

   _____

   _____

   b. Special purpose computer: _____

   _____

   _____

   c. Byte: _____

   _____

   _____

   d. Output device: _____

   _____

   _____

   e. Computer software: _____

   _____

   _____

   f. Programming language: _____

   _____

   _____

   g. Personal computer: _____

   _____

   _____

h. IBM clone: _____

_____

_____

i. Cursor: _____

_____

_____

j. Drive C: _____

_____

_____

k. Printout: _____

_____

_____

l. Operating system: _____

_____

_____

m. File: _____

_____

_____

n. Network: _____

_____

_____

o. Communications software: _____

_____

_____

p. Coding: _____

_____

_____

q. Missing data: _____

_____

_____

r. Fixed format: _____

_____

_____

s. Free format: _____

_____

_____

t. Right-justification: _____

_____

_____

u. Field: _____

_____

_____

v. Edge-coding: _____

_____

_____

w. Outlier: _____

_____

_____

x. Consistency check: _____

_____

_____

y. Codebook: _____

_____

_____

2. Examine Figure 20-3 in the textbook. Describe in your own words the flow of operations for processing the data and commands from the 30 subjects described in the "Using a Packaged Program" section. Indicate specific I/O devices that might be used.

3. Complete the codebook that is started in Figure 20-8 (based on questions 5 through 11 of Figure 20-7).

D. Application Exercises

1. Kenneally,* a student researcher, was learning to prepare SPSS-PC instructions to analyze her data. The data consisted of information for the following variables: subject's age, smoking status (smoker/nonsmoker), and number of days absent from work during 1990. A total of 125 men and women provided data for this study. Below are the SPSS instructions that Kenneally initially prepared to obtain basic descriptive statistics, such as frequency counts (e.g., number of smokers in her sample):

   ```
   DATA LIST
     /AGE 1 SMOKESTATUS 2 DAYSABSNT 3.
   FREQUENCIES = AGE, SMOKESTATUS, DAYSABSNT
     /STATISTICS = ALL.
   BEGIN DATA.
   ```

   There are five errors in this set of instructions. Make the necessary changes to remove the errors.

2. Newey†, a student researcher, developed a preliminary coding layout for her questionnaire (which focused on the postgraduation experiences of nursing school students). A portion of that layout is presented on the following page, together with Newey's plans for coding missing data. Review and critique the coding layout on the next page. Suggest improvements that you feel are needed. To assist you in your critique, here are some guiding questions:

   a. What is the maximum number of respondents that the coding scheme allows?

   b. Check the field width for each question. Are extra columns needed to code all possible responses? Are there too many columns allocated for some questions?

   c. Examine the coding categories specified for the precoded questions. Are they reasonable and consistent? Do they permit all responses to be adequately coded?

   d. Examine the missing data codes and comment on their appropriateness. Does the researcher distinguish between different types of missing data? If not, should she have? Do any of the missing codes conflict with actual codes? Recommend changes as necessary.

   e. When you have made all the changes you believe are needed (if any), how many columns in total will be required to include all the data produced for these 10 questions?

---

*This example is fictitious.

†This example is fictitious. The example was not intended to reflect proper sequencing or distribution of questionnaire items, but was designed to include points covered in the text related to coding.

TO BE ENTERED IN COLUMNS	MISSING VALUES CODE	QUESTION
1–4		ID Number

5	9	1. Are you currently employed?
		  1. yes
		  2. no (SKIP TO Q 7)

6	9	2. How many hours do you work in a typical week? _____
7–10	9	3. What is your monthly salary? $ _____

11	9	4. In what type of setting are you currently employed?
		  1. hospital or clinic
		  2. nursing home
		  3. school
		  4. private practice
		  5. community agency
		  6. health-maintenance organization
		  7. industry
		  8. other nursing-related settings
		  9. other non-nursing-related settings

12–13	9	5. How many other nurses are employed by the same agency/institution that employs you? _____

14	9	6. How satisfied are you with your present position?
		  1. very satisfied
		  2. somewhat satisfied
		  3. neither satisfied nor dissatisfied
		  4. somewhat dissatisfied
		  5. very dissatisfied
		    (SKIP TO Q 9)

15	9	7. Are you currently seeking employment?
		  1. yes
		  2. no (SKIP TO Q 9)

16	9	8. Which of the following have you done in trying to find a job?
		  1. read newspaper ads
		  2. contacted my school's placement office
		  3. gone to an employment agency
		  4. called or written to institutions directly
		  5. called employed friends to see if they knew of any openings

17–18	9	9. How old are you? _____

19	9	10. What is your marital status?
		  1. single, never married
		  2. married
		  3. separated or divorced
		  4. widowed

E. Special Projects

1. Visit a computer center and ask for a tour of the mainframe hardware facilities. Make a list of the I/O devices available to users. Make a list of the statistical software packages available.

2. As indicated throughout the text, research primarily focuses on the relationships between variables. For instance, in the example presented in the Application Exercise (D.1), the researcher would probably be interested in learning if the average number of days absent is higher among smokers than nonsmokers. The SPSS command for this computation is as follows:

   MEANS TABLES = VARX BY VARY.

   where VARX is the continuous dependent variable (here, number of days absent) and VARY is the categorical independent variable (smoking status).

   Suppose that you were interested in studying birth outcomes in various groups of women. Suppose further that you have collected data from 150 women who have just given birth, with respect to the following variables: age group (under 20/20 and over); birthweight of infant (in ounces); Apgar score (from 1 to 10); ethnicity of mother (white/black/Hispanic); and type of delivery (vaginal/cesarean). Write out SPSS instructions that would (a) produce frequency information for these five variables; (b) compare the birthweights in the two age groups; and (c) compare the Apgar scores for the two types of delivery.

3. Ask 10 to 15 of your friends to respond to the following question:

   What is the *one* least satisfying aspect about being a nurse, in your opinion?

   Develop codes for this question based on the themes expressed in the responses you obtain. Compare your coding scheme with that prepared by other fellow students.

Chapter 21

DESIGNING AND IMPLEMENTING AN ANALYSIS STRATEGY

A. *Matching Exercises*

Match each phrase from Set B with one (or more) of the missing values strategies listed in Set A. Indicate the letter(s) corresponding to your response next to each of the statements in Set B.

SET A

a. Listwise deletion
b. Deletion of variable
c. Mean substitution
d. Estimation of missing value
e. Pairwise deletion

SET B   RESPONSE

1. Complete deletion of missing cases   _____

2. Results in a nonrectangular matrix   _____

3. Multiple regression can be used to achieve this   _____

4. Useful when there are missing values for a few items on a
   scale   _____

5. Not an attractive option when the missing values are on a key
   variable   _____

6. Not an attractive option when the sample size is very small _____

Polit DF, Hungler BP: STUDY GUIDE FOR NURSING RESEARCH:
PRINCIPLES AND METHODS, 5th ed. © 1995 J.B. Lippincott Company.

7. Usually more precise than mean substitution   _____
8. A good solution if a subject has extensive missing data   _____
9. Results in a sample that is a "moving target"   _____
10. Useful when there is missing data on a variable for a high percentage of subjects   _____

B. Completion Exercises

Write the words or phrases that correctly complete the sentences below.

1. It is almost inevitable for a data set to have some _____ _____ , creating potential problems that the researcher must address.

2. If men had significantly more missing information than women on a question about their use of illegal drugs, this would indicate the presence of _____ _____ .

3. If a data set had data values for all subjects on all variables, the data set would be a _____ _____ of data.

4. Raw data often need to be _____ _____ or altered before proceeding to statistical analysis.

5. When an item on a 7-point scale is changed from a value of 2 to a value of 6, this is called a(n) _____ _____ .

6. Researchers collecting data from several sites often perform tests to determine if the data can be _____ _____ .

7. When data are voluminous, researchers sometimes develop _____ _____ to guide the analysis of data.

8. In quantitative studies, the statistical analyses yield the _____ _____ of the study.

9. The first step in the interpretation of research findings involves an analysis of the

_____

____ of the results, based on various types of evidence.

10. It is useful for a researcher to perform a _____ _____ when the results of the main hypothesis tests were not statistically significant.

11. In quantitative analysis, the results are generally in the form of _____ _____ and _____ .

12. Interpretation of results is easiest when the results are consistent with the researcher's _____ _____ .

13. Because researchers are not generally interested in discovering relationships exclusively for the research sample, an important part of the interpretive process involves an assessment of the _____ _____ of the results.

14. An important research precept is that _____ _____ does not prove causation.

15. Nonsignificant findings mean that the null hypothesis is _____ _____ ; significant findings mean that the null hypothesis is _____ _____ .

C. Study Questions

1. Define the following terms. Compare your definition with the definition in Chapter 21 of the textbook or in the glossary.

   a. Listwise deletion: _____

   _____

   _____

b. Pairwise deletion: _____

_____

_____

c. Dummy variable: _____

_____

_____

d. Recoded data: _____

_____

_____

e. Ceiling effect: _____

_____

_____

f. Manipulation check: _____

_____

_____

g. Cohort effect: _____

_____

_____

h. Negative results: _____

_____

_____

i. Positive results: _____

_____

_____

j. Mixed results: _____

_____

_____

2. Write out the SPSS instructions to create a composite variable called ATTITUDE, based on the questions shown in Table 13-3 of the textbook. Remember to reverse the negatively worded questions.

3. Write out the SPSS instructions to create dichotomous variables for ANXIETY and SUPRATING (anxiety scores and supervisor's performance ratings), for the data presented in Exercise E.1 in Chapter 17 in this *Study Guide*. Use the median of these two variables (which you will need to compute) to dichotomize the variables.

4. Create a table shell for displaying some statistical analyses using the data presented in Exercise E.1 in Chapter 17 of this *Study Guide*.

5. Below are several suggested research articles in which the researchers obtained mixed results—that is, some hypotheses were supported, and others were not. Review and critique the researchers' interpretation of the findings for one or more of these studies and suggest some possible alternatives.

   • DiIorio, C., Faherty, B., & Manteuffel, B. (1994). Epilepsy self-management: Partial replication and extension. *Research in Nursing and Health, 17,* 167–174.

   • Lierman, L. M., Young, H. M., Powell-Cope, G., Georgiadou, F., & Benoliel, J. Q. (1994). Effects of education and support on breast self-examination in older women. *Nursing Research, 43,* 158–163.

   • Miller, K. M., & Perry, P. A. (1990). Relaxation technique and postoperative pain in patients undergoing cardiac surgery. *Heart and Lung, 19,* 136–146.

   • Naylor, M. D. (1990). Comprehensive discharge planning for hospitalized elderly: A pilot study. *Nursing Research, 39,* 156–161.

D. Application Exercise

1. Coulter and Kelley (1995)* studied the relationship between marital quality during pregnancy and postpartum depression in a sample of couples expecting their first child. Data on marital satisfaction, perceived relationship quality, and egalitarianism of marital roles were gathered during the second trimester of the pregnancy from 157 couples (157 women and 116 men completed three scales and demographic forms). Information on birth outcomes were available for 149 infants. Maternal depression was measured 2 weeks after delivery for 138 mothers. Here are some of the things that the researchers decided to do before they conducted their substantive analyses:

   • Use data for only the 110 families for which there was data for all three types of information (male and female partners' marital data; birth outcomes; and maternal depression).

   • Compute the reliability (internal consistency) of the three marital quality scales, separately for men and women.

   • Analyze differences between the men who did and did not complete the predelivery information (in terms of their partner's background characteristics and perceptions of marital quality).

*This example is fictitious.

- Analyze differences between the women who agreed to complete the depression scale postpartum and those who did not (in terms of own and their partner's background characteristics and perceptions of marital quality, and birth outcomes).

Review and comment on these decisions. Suggest alternative and additional preanalysis activities for the researchers. To aid you in this task, here are some guiding questions:

  a. Did the researchers handle missing data problems in the most effective manner? What other approaches might have been used? What are the consequences of the alternative strategies?

  b. How did the researchers evaluate data quality? Was this an appropriate strategy? What other steps could have been taken to ensure high-quality data?

  c. What did the researchers do to evaluate bias? Was this an appropriate strategy? What other methods could have been used to examine bias?

  d. What (if any) additional analyses should the researchers have undertaken before addressing the main substantive analyses?

2. Below are several suggested research articles. Read one of these articles and respond (to the extent possible) to questions a through d from Question D.1 with regard to this actual research study.

   - Griffin, C., Dougherty, M. C., & Yarandi, H. (1994). Pelvic muscles during rest: Responses to pelvic muscle exercise. *Nursing Research, 43,* 164–167.
   - Hill, P. D., & Aldag, J. C. (1993). Insufficient milk supply among black and white breast-feeding mothers. *Research in Nursing and Health, 16,* 203–211.
   - Kim, M. J., Larson, J. L., Covey, M. K., Vitalo, C. A., Alex, C. G., & Patel, M. (1993). Inspiratory muscle training in patients with chronic obstructive pulmonary disease. *Nursing Research, 42,* 356–361.
   - Woods, N. F., Lentz, M. J., Mitchell, E. S., & Kogan, H. (1994). Arousal and stress response across the menstrual cycle in women with three perimenstrual symptom patterns. *Research in Nursing and Health, 17,* 99–110.

E. Special Projects

1. Read one of the studies listed in Question D.2 of this chapter. Compare your interpretation of the results with the interpretation of the researchers, as presented in the Discussion section of the report.

2. Based on the table presented in Question D.1 of Chapter 18 of this *Study Guide,* prepare a written discussion of the results of Wells' study.

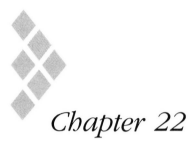

Chapter 22

THE ANALYSIS OF
QUALITATIVE DATA

A. Matching Exercises

Match each descriptive statement from Set B with one (or more) of the statements from Set A. Indicate the letter(s) corresponding to your response next to each item in Set B.

SET A
a. Analytic induction approach
b. Grounded theory approach
c. Qualitative content analysis
d. None of the above

SET B   RESPONSE

1. Can be facilitated through use of computers   _____
2. Involves the technique known as constant comparison _____
3. Typically involves quantification   _____
4. Involves the development of an inductively derived hypothesis   _____
5. Involves the analysis of narrative materials   _____
6. Requires data saturation   _____
7. Can be used in ethnographic studies   _____
8. Requires data to be categorized and coded   _____
9. Can be used to collect psychological data   _____
10. Alternates between tentative explanation and definition _____

Polit DF, Hungler BP: STUDY GUIDE FOR NURSING RESEARCH:
PRINCIPLES AND METHODS, 5th ed. © 1995 J.B. Lippincott Company.

B. *Completion Exercises*

Write the words or phrases that correctly complete the sentences below.

1. The term *holistic* is more often used to describe _____

    _____ than _____

    _____ research.

2. In qualitative research, hypothesis _____

    _____ is frequently a goal.

3. The task in organizing qualitative data is to develop a mechanism to _____

    _____ the data.

4. Typically, a qualitative researcher develops a comprehensive _____

    _____ scheme for

    coding the data.

5. When data are organized manually, researchers usually insert excerpts of the data

    into _____

    _____ .

6. Most qualitative data management programs require that a word processing file

    be imported in _____

    _____ format.

7. The analysis of qualitative data generally begins with a search for _____

    _____ .

8. The use of _____

    _____ involves an accounting of the frequency with which certain

    themes and relationships are supported by the data.

9. The approach known as _____

    _____ involves an interactive process in which qualitative

    data are used to pose questions and arrive at tentative explanations.

10. The approach known as _____

    _____ involves a constant comparative approach to col-

    lecting and analyzing qualitative data, with an eye toward theory development.

11. Hermeneutic analysis is associated with _____

_____ research.

12. Research that focuses on cognitive processes as expressed verbally may involve

the application of _____

_____ .

C. Study Questions

1. Define the following terms. Compare your definition with the definition in Chapter 22 of the textbook or in the glossary.

a. Qualitative analysis: _____

_____

_____

b. Administrative files: _____

_____

_____

c. Conceptual files: _____

_____

_____

d. Quasi-statistics: _____

_____

_____

e. Grounded theory: _____

_____

_____

f. Data saturation: _____

_____

_____

g. Constant comparison: _____

_____

_____

2. For each of the problem statements below, indicate whether you think a researcher should collect primarily qualitative or quantitative data. Justify your response.

a. How do victims of AIDS cope with the discovery of their illness? _____

_____

_____

b. What important dimensions of nursing practice differ in developed and underdeveloped countries? _____

_____

_____

c. What is the effect of therapeutic touch on patient well-being? _____

_____

_____

d. Do nurse practitioners and physicians differ in the performance of triage functions? _____

_____

_____

e. Is a patient's length of stay in hospital related to the quality or quantity of his or her social supports? _____

_____

_____

f. How does the typical American feel about such new reproductive technologies as in vitro fertilization? _____

_____

_____

g. What are the psychological sequelae of having an organ transplantation? ___

_____

_____

h. By what processes do women make decisions about having amniocentesis?

_____

_____

i. What factors are most predictive of a woman giving birth to a very-low-birthweight infant? _____

_____

_____

j. What effects does caffeine have on gastrointestinal motility? _____

_____

_____

3. A category scheme for coding interviews with recently divorced women follows:

CODING SCHEME FOR STUDY OF ADJUSTMENT TO DIVORCE

1. Divorce-related issues
   a. Adjustment to divorce
   b. Divorce-induced problems
   c. Advantages of divorce
2. General psychologic state
   a. Before divorce
   b. During divorce
   c. Current
3. Physical health
   a. Before divorce
   b. During divorce
   c. Current
4. Relationship with children
   a. General quality
   b. Communication
   c. Shared activities
   d. Structure of relationship
5. Parenting
   a. Discipline and child-rearing

(continued)

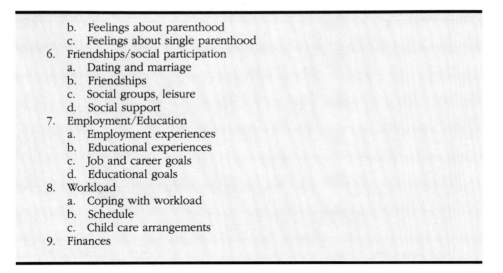

b. Feelings about parenthood
c. Feelings about single parenthood
6. Friendships/social participation
    a. Dating and marriage
    b. Friendships
    c. Social groups, leisure
    d. Social support
7. Employment/Education
    a. Employment experiences
    b. Educational experiences
    c. Job and career goals
    d. Educational goals
8. Workload
    a. Coping with workload
    b. Schedule
    c. Child care arrangements
9. Finances

Read the following excerpt, taken from a real interview. Use the coding scheme to code the topics discussed in this excerpt.

I think raising the children is so much easier without the father around. There isn't two people conflicting back and forth. You know, like . . . like you discipline them during the day. They do something wrong, you're not saying, "When daddy gets home, you're going to get a spanking." You know, you do that. The kid gets a spanking right then and there. But when two people live together, they have their ways of raising and you have your ways of raising the children and it's so hard for two people to raise children. It's so much easier for one person. The only reason a male would be around is financial-wise. But me and the kids are happier now, and we get along with each other better, cause like, there isn't this competitive thing. My husband always wanted all the attention around here.

D. Application Exercises

1. Sarno (1995)* studied the phenomenon of "being on precautions" from the perspective of hospitalized adults. She began her study, after securing permission, by spending 2 days on the hospital units where the data would be collected. The 2 days were spent familiarizing herself with the units, learning how best to collect the data, determining where she could position herself in an unobtrusive manner, and establishing a trusting relationship with the nursing staff.

*This example is fictitious.

The data for the study were collected using the techniques of observation and unstructured interviewing. Sarno selectively sampled all times of the day and all days of the week in 2-hour segments to make her observations. The time schedule began on a Monday morning at 7:00 AM and continued until 9:00 AM. On Tuesday, the observation time became 9:00 AM until 11:00 AM. Observations continued around the clock on consecutive days until no new information was being collected. Sarno either positioned herself directly outside the door to the patient's room or sat in the patient's room to make her observations. Observations included any activity or interaction between the patient and hospital staff or between the patient and Sarno.

The unstructured interviewing process consisted of asking patients to clarify why they were doing certain things and what they liked or disliked about the hospital experience.

Sarno recorded the observations and data from the interviews in a log immediately after each 2-hour observation segment. All data were recorded in chronologic order. Sarno also recorded any feelings she had during the observation experience. As time progressed, she reread her field notes after every 4 hours of observation. As commonalities began to emerge from the data, she developed another section to her log according to similarity of content and referenced the daily log notes according to commonalities. Sarno continued making observations until she thought she had a "feel for the data" and that additional observations or interactions provided only redundant information. A total of five patients were observed.

Categories that emerged from the data were labeled "avoidance," "devaluation as a person," and "loneliness." Evidence for the avoidance perspective came from patient comments during informal conversations with the researcher and the observational field notes. The evidence included statements such as, "Nurses seldom come into the room because they have to put all that [pointing to precaution gowns] stuff on"; "Look, she [the cleaning woman] won't come in the room. She's afraid of me"; "Did you see that? Only my doctor would touch me. The rest were afraid to touch me." Observational field notes contained several notations of nurses coming to the door of the room asking, "Do you want anything?" but not entering the room.

The category "devaluation as a person" emerged from comments such as, "I don't like being treated as a specimen"; "Do you have to wear gloves every time you take care of me [made to a nurse]?"; "If I go to the door of the room, they [the nurses] yell at me [made to the researcher]."

The category "loneliness" was developed from field notes that observed patients occasionally putting the call light on to find out what time it was or how long until lunch, or asking about a noise they had heard. Comments that conveyed the same feeling of loneliness were, "Being confined in this room is like being in jail"; "I can't wait to get out of here and have dinner with my friends"; and "The hours seem endless here."

Review and critique this study. Suggest alternative ways of collecting and analyzing the data for the research problem. To assist you in your critique, here are some guiding questions:

a. Comment on the choice of research approach. Was a qualitative research approach suitable for the phenomenon being studied? In your opinion, would a more quantitative research approach have been more appropriate?

b. The data in the study were collected by observation and informal interviewing. Could the data have been collected in another way? Should they have been?

c. What type of sampling plan was used to sample observations in the study? Would an alternative sampling plan have been better? Why or why not?

d. The researcher recorded her observations, feelings, and interviews immediately after each 2-hour observation period. Comment on the appropriateness of this method. Can you identify any biases that could be present in this choice of method? Suggest alternative ways of recording the data.

e. Categorize the field notes made in the study according to their purpose. What additional types of field notes would you have included?

f. How did the researcher handle the concept of theoretical saturation? Could you recommend any improvements?

g. What types of validation procedures did the researcher use? Can you suggest additional procedures that might have improved the study?

h. Comment on the categories that emerged from the data. Do they appear to reflect accurately the data that were collected? Would you have developed different ones?

2. Below are several suggested research articles. Skim one or more of these articles and respond to questions a through h from Question D.1, to the extent possible, in terms of the actual research study.

- Bailey, B. J., & Kahn, A. (1993). Apportioning illness management authority: How diabetic individuals evaluate and respond to spousal help. *Qualitative Health Research, 3,* 55–73.
- Dick, M. J. (1993). Preterm infants in pain. *Clinical Nursing Research, 2,* 176–187.
- May, K. A. (1994). Impact of maternal activity restriction for preterm labor on the expectant father. *Journal of Obstetric, Gynecologic, and Neonatal Nursing, 23,* 246–252.
- Pinch, W. J., & Spielman, M. L. (1993). Parental perceptions of ethical issues post-NICU discharge. *Western Journal of Nursing Research, 15,* 422–437.
- Rather, M. L. (1992). "Nursing as a way of thinking"—Heideggerian hermeneutical analysis of the lived experience of the returning RN. *Research in Nursing and Health, 15,* 47–56.

- Stevens, P. E. (1994). Protective strategies of lesbian clients in health care environments. *Research in Nursing and Health, 17,* 217–230.
- Swanson, J. M., & Chenitz, W. C. (1993). Regaining a valued self: The process of adaptation to living with genital herpes. *Qualitative Health Research, 3,* 270–297.

E. Special Projects

1. Get 10 or so people to write one or two paragraphs on their feelings about death and dying. Perform a thematic analysis of these paragraphs.

2. Develop two or three research questions that you think might lend themselves to a qualitative study.

3. Read one of the studies listed in the Suggested Readings section of Chapter 22 in the textbook. Generate several hypotheses that could be tested based on the reported findings.

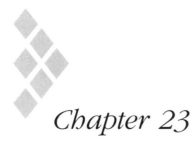

Chapter 23

INTEGRATION OF QUALITATIVE AND QUANTITATIVE ANALYSIS

A. Matching Exercises

Match each descriptive statement from Set B with one of the statements from Set A. Indicate the letter corresponding to your response next to each item in Set B.

SET A
a. Qualitative data
b. Quantitative data
c. Both qualitative and quantitative data
d. Neither qualitative nor quantitative data

SET B   RESPONSE

1. Should be collected to help improve nursing practice   _____
2. Are especially useful for understanding dynamic processes   _____
3. Are often collected in large-scale surveys   _____
4. Are useful in *proving* the validity of theories   _____
5. Are usually collected by phenomenological researchers   _____
6. Can profit from triangulation   _____
7. Are often used in tests of causal relationships   _____
8. Can contribute to theoretical insights   _____

9. Require validity checks   _____

10. Tend to be collected from small samples   _____

B. Completion Exercises

Write the words or phrases that correctly complete the sentences below.

1. Qualitative and quantitative data may, for some research problems, be _____

_____ in

that they "mutually supply each other's lack."

2. The major conceptual frameworks of nursing demand neither _____

_____ nor _____ data.

3. Progress in a developing area of research tends to be _____

_____ and can profit from

multiple feedback loops.

4. A major advantage of integrating different approaches is potential enhancements

to the study's _____

_____ .

5. A frequent application of integration is in the development of research _____

_____

6. In a quantitative study, the inclusion of qualitative data might facilitate the

_____

_____ of the findings, and vice versa.

7. When qualitative data collection is embedded in a survey effort, it is often more

productive to use a _____

_____ approach.

8. In studies of the effects of complex interventions, qualitative data may be useful

in addressing the _____

_____ question.

9. A major barrier to integration is _____

_____ biases.

10. Although an integrated data collection and analysis approach is _____

_____ , it can be ar-

gued that the collection of multiple types of data in a single study is efficient.

C. Study Questions

1. Define the following terms. Compare your definition with the definition in Chapter 23 of the textbook or in the glossary.

   a. Multimethod research: _____

   _____

   _____

   b. Black box: _____

   _____

   _____

   c. Epistemological bias: _____

   _____

   _____

   d. Complementarity: _____

   _____

   _____

2. Read one of the following studies, in which qualitative data were gathered and analyzed to address a research question. Suggest ways in which the collection of quantitative data might have enriched the study, strengthened its validity, and/or enhanced its interpretability:

   - Aroian, K. J. (1992). Sources of social support and conflict for Polish immigrants. *Qualitative Health Research, 2,* 178–207.
   - Fisher, B. J., & Peterson, C. (1993). She won't be dancing much anyway: A study of surgeons, surgical nurses, and elderly patients. *Qualitative Health Research, 3,* 165–183.
   - Hamera, E. K., Pallikkathayil, L., Bauer, S., & Burton, M. R. (1994). Descriptions of wellness by individuals with schizophrenia. *Western Journal of Nursing Research, 16,* 268–287.

- Karp, D. A. (1994). Living with depression: Illness and identity turning points. *Qualitative Health Research, 4,* 6–30.
- McBride, S. (1993). Perceived control in patients with chronic obstructive pulmonary disease. *Western Journal of Nursing Research, 15,* 456–464.

3. Read one of the following studies, in which quantitative data were gathered and analyzed to address a research question. Suggest ways in which the collection of qualitative data might have enriched the study, strengthened its validity, or enhanced its interpretability:

- Ailinger, R. L., Dear, M. R., & Holley-Wilcox, P. (1993). Predictors of function among older Hispanic immigrants: A five-year follow-up study. *Nursing Research, 42,* 240–244.
- Brown, M. A., & Lewis, L. L. (1993). Cycle-phase changes in perceived stress in women with varying levels of premenstrual symptomatology. *Research in Nursing and Health, 16,* 423–429.
- Hall, C., & Lanig, H. (1993). Spiritual caring behaviors as reported by Christian nurses. *Western Journal of Nursing Research, 15,* 730–741.
- Prattke, T. W., & Gass-Sternas, K. A. (1993). Appraisal, coping, and emotional health of infertile couples undergoing donor artificial insemination. *Journal of Gynecologic, Obstetric, and Neonatal Nursing, 22,* 516–527.
- Reinhard, S. C. (1994). Living with mental illness: Effects of professional support and personal control on caregiver burden. *Research in Nursing and Health, 17,* 79–88.

D. Application Exercises

1. Zack (1995)* conducted a study to investigate breastfeeding practices among teenaged mothers, who have been found in many studies to be less likely than older mothers to breastfeed. Using birth records from two large hospitals, Zack contacted 250 young women between 15 and 19 years of age who had given birth in the previous year and invited them to participate in a survey. Those who agreed to participate ($N = 185$) were interviewed by telephone (when possible), using a structured interview that asked about breastfeeding practices, attitudes toward motherhood, availability of social supports, and conflicting demands, such as school attendance or employment. Several psychological scales (including measures of depression and self-esteem) were also administered. Teenagers without a telephone were interviewed in person in their own homes. All the teenagers interviewed at home were also interviewed in greater depth, using a topic guide that focused on such areas as feelings about breastfeeding, the decision-making process that led them to decide whether or not to breastfeed, barriers to breastfeeding, and intentions to breastfeed with any subsequent chil-

*This study is fictitious.

dren. Zack used the quantitative data to determine the characteristics associated with breastfeeding status and duration. The qualitative data were used to interpret and validate the quantitative findings.

Review and critique this study. Suggest alternative data collection and analysis approaches. To assist you in your critique, here are some guiding questions:

a. Which of the aims of integration, if any, were served by this study?

b. What was the researcher's basic strategy for integration? How effective was this strategy in addressing the aims of integration?

c. Suggest ways of altering the design of the study and the data collection approach to further promote integrative aims.

d. Would the study have been stronger if it had involved the collection of quantitative data only? Qualitative data only? Why or why not?

2. Below are several suggested research articles of studies that used an integrated approach. Read one or more of these articles and respond to questions a through d from Question D.1 in terms of these actual research studies.

- Carrieri, V. K., Kieckhefer, G., Janson-Bjerklie, S., & Souza, J. (1991). The sensation of pulmonary dyspnea in school-age children. *Nursing Research, 40,* 81–85.

- Halm, M. A., Titler, M. G., Kleiber, C., Johnson, S. K., Montgomery, L. A., Craft, M. J., Buckwalter, K., Nicholson, A., & Megivern, K. (1993). Behavioral responses of family members during critical illness. *Clinical Nursing Research, 2,* 414–437.

- Lev, E. L. (1992). Patients' strategies for adapting to cancer treatment. *Western Journal of Nursing Research, 14,* 595–612.

- Long, K. A., & Weinert, C. (1992). Descriptions and perceptions of health among rural and urban adults with multiple sclerosis. *Research in Nursing and Health, 15,* 335–342.

- Smith, C. E., Mayer, L. S., Parkhurst, C., Perkins, S. B., & Pingleton, S. K. (1991). Adaptation in families with a member requiring mechanical ventilation at home. *Heart and Lung, 20,* 349–356.

E. Special Projects

1. Prepare five problem statements that would be amenable to multimethod research.

2. For one of the problems suggested in Exercise E.1, write a two- to three-page description of how the data would be collected and how the use of both qualitative and quantitative data and analysis would strengthen the study.

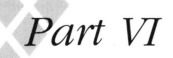

Part VI

COMMUNICATION IN THE RESEARCH PROCESS

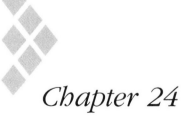

Chapter 24

WRITING A RESEARCH REPORT

A. Matching Exercises

Match each sentence from Set B with one of the sections in a research report in which these sentences would appear, as listed in Set A. Indicate the letter corresponding to your response next to each of the statements in Set B.

SET A
a. Introduction
b. Methods section
c. Results section
d. Discussion section

SET B   **RESPONSE**

1. The sample consisted of 50 men aged 65 to 75 years, selected at random from a nursing home.   _____

2. These data suggest that nurses have become increasingly less accepting of traditional sex-role stereotypes.   _____

3. It is hypothesized that male and female paraplegics differ in their perceptions of the importance of architectural barriers.   _____

4. The 100 subjects were randomly assigned to the experimental and control groups using a random-numbers table.   _____

5. Mothers who breastfed their babies were significantly more likely than those who did not to express favorable views toward the motherhood role ($t = 3.22$, $df = 98$, $p < .01$).   _____

6. A major flaw of studies conducted to date is the low reliability of the instruments the researchers used.   _____

7. The findings reported here are consistent with the work of Hogan (1990) and Crimmins (1988), both of whom used as subjects patients with MI.   _____

8. Age at marriage was found to be significantly related to both educational attainment ($r = -.25$) and number of children ($r = -.38$).   _____

B. Completion Exercises

Write the words or phrases that correctly complete the sentences below.

1. The _____

   _____ section of a report discusses the researcher's aims, the research questions, and the context of the study.

2. The _____

   _____ section of a report describes what the researcher did to gather and analyze the data.

3. Research findings are described in the _____

   _____ section of a report.

4. Statistical information can most effectively and succinctly be displayed in _____

   _____ .

5. Graphic presentations of statistical information are usually referred to as _____

   _____ .

6. Interpretations of results are normally presented in the _____

   _____ section of a report.

7. The main communication outlet for scholarly research activity is _____

   _____ .

8. When a research report is authored by more than one person who made equal contributions, the names are listed _____

   _____ .

C. Study Questions

1. Define the following terms. Compare your definition with the definition in Chapter 24 of the textbook or in the glossary.

   a. Research report: _____

   _____

   _____

   b. Summary: _____

   _____

   _____

   c. Journal article: _____

   _____

   _____

   d. Blind review: _____

   _____

   _____

   e. Call for papers: _____

   _____

   _____

   f. Poster session: _____

   _____

   _____

   g. Refereed journal: _____

   _____

   _____

2. The following sentences all have stylistic flaws. Suggest ways in which the sentences could be improved.

   a. ICU nurses experience more stress than nurses on a general ward ($t = 2.5$, $df = 148$, $p < .05$)

   _____

   _____

b. "A Study Investigating the Effect of Primary Care Nursing on the Emotional Well-Being of Patients in a Cardiac Care Unit."

_____

_____

c. The nonsignificant results demonstrate that there is no relationship between diet and hyperkinesis.

_____

_____

d. It has, therefore, been proved that people have a more negative body image if the age of onset of obesity is before age 20 years.

_____

_____

e. The positive significant relationship indicates that occupational stress causes sleep disturbances.

_____

_____

3. Suppose that you were the author of a research article with the titles indicated below. For each, name two different journals to which your article could be submitted for publication.

a. "Parental attachment to children with Down's syndrome." _____

_____

_____

b. "Sexual functioning among men in their 70s." _____

_____

_____

c. "Comparison of therapists' and clients' expectations regarding psychiatric therapy." _____

_____

_____

d. "The effects of fetal monitoring on selected birth outcomes." _____

_____

_____

e. "Effectiveness of alternative methods of relieving pressure sores." _____

_____

_____

4. Suggest titles for five of the fictitious studies described in the Application sections of this study guide.

5. Suppose you were studying the psychological well-being of women who had just experienced a miscarriage in comparison of women who were still pregnant in the second month of their pregnancy. For these two groups, the mean scores, respectively, on four scales are 15.1 and 10.7 (depression); 23.6 and 23.9 (mood); 17.9 and 15.7 (marital satisfaction); and 18.9 and 25.8 (self-efficacy). Prepare a table to display these results. (Embellish the table by inventing either standard deviation information or results of t-tests).

D. *Application Exercises*

1. Israel (1995)* hypothesized that preschool children from single-parent families are more likely than those from two-parent families to display negative behavioral and psychosocial patterns. She administered a behavioral checklist to 30 divorced mothers and 30 married mothers who accompanied their preschool child (3–5 years of age) during immunization for measles. Each mother was asked to indicate the frequency with which these preschool children exhibited a series of behaviors ("very often," "fairly often," "sometimes," or "never"). Examples of the behavioral items include, "often cries with little or no apparent reason," "tends to sulk when unable to have his or her own way," and "has trouble making or keeping friends." The items were combined to form three subscales: Home and Family; Friends and Peers; and General. A total Behavioral Adjustment score was also computed. The table below presents the results:

	ONE-PARENT Means*	TWO-PARENT Means*	t	p
Home and family	17.5	16.8	1.5	>.05
Friends and Peers	19.1	19.4	0.9	>.05
General Behaviors	24.7	25.3	1.1	>.05
Overall Behavioral Adjustment	61.3	61.5	0.7	>.05

*Higher scores reflect *better* adjustment.

Here is how Israel described her results:

Contrary to expectations, the behavioral patterns of the children from intact and one-parent homes were very similar. With respect to Home and Family behaviors, in fact, children in the one-parent homes were superior. Friendship patterns and interactions with peers were virtually identical in the two groups. In terms of general behaviors, such as crying, pouting, or acting out, the children from the two-parent families showed a slight edge. Overall, the two groups performed about equivalently. Thus, it may be concluded that preschool children who live in one-parent families are not handicapped by the absence of their fathers. Their behaviors are normal and not different from those of their same-aged peers from intact homes. In one area, children from the one-parent home show evidence of more favorable behaviors than those with both parents at home.

Review and critique the above description. Suggest alternative ways of describing and interpreting the results. To help you in your critique, here are some guiding questions:

    a. Comment on the content of the excerpt. Did the author omit discussing any important results? Was there any redundancy—could the summary have been more succinct?

    b. Comment on the accuracy of the report. Does the text agree with the table? Does the report imply statistically significant results that were in fact not in the data?

    c. Comment on the style of the report. Does the author use language that is too subjective? Does the author fail to use language that is in keeping with the tentative nature of research? Does the author use jargon or unnecessary technical terms?

    d. Comment on the author's interpretation of the results. Does the author read too much into the data? Does the author suggest several possible explanations for the findings? In the interpretation, does the author try to take into consideration such factors as the smallness of the sample, the influence of extraneous variables, inadequacies of the measuring instrument, and so on?

2. Below are several suggested research articles. Skim one (or more) of these articles, focusing especially on the researcher's results and discussion sections. Respond to questions a through d from Question D.1 in terms of the actual research study.

- Grace, J. T. (1993). Mothers' self-reports of parenthood across the first 6 months postpartum. *Research in Nursing and Health, 16,* 431–439.

- Haq, M. B. (1993). Understanding older adult satisfaction with primary health care services at a nursing center. *Applied Nursing Research, 6,* 125–131.

- Jablonski, R. S. (1994). The experience of being mechanically ventilated. *Qualitative Health Research, 4,* 186–207.

- Meier, P. P., Engstrom, J. L., Mangurten, H. H., Estrada, E., Zimmerman, B., & Kopparthi, R. (1993). Breastfeeding support services in the neonatal intensive care unit. *Journal of Obstetric, Gynecologic, and Neonatal Nursing, 22,* 338–347.

- Simington, J. A., & Laing, G. P. (1993). Effects of therapeutic touch on anxiety in the institutionalized elderly. *Clinical Nursing Research, 2,* 438–451.

E. Special Projects

1. Suppose that you were studying maternal behavior in mothers of normal and handicapped children. Fifty mothers from each group are observed interacting with their children (7–10 years of age) in a laboratory setting for 30 minutes. Some data are presented below:

MEAN NO. OF:	*MOTHERS WITH NORMAL CHILDREN*	*MOTHERS WITH HANDICAPPED CHILDREN*	*t*
Times mother initiates conversations	10.2	12.8	2.3
Minutes of silence	14.9	13.8	1.7
Times mother laughs or smiles	8.4	7.9	1.2
Direct maternal commands	8.7	6.1	3.8
Encouraging or supportive comments	4.1	5.7	2.4

Write a brief Results and Discussion section for these data.

2. Read the article, "Coping with cancer," by Kaisa Krause, which appeared in the *Western Journal of Nursing Research,* 1993, Vol. 15, pages 31–40. Prepare an abstract for this study.

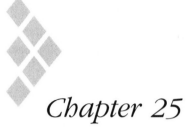

Chapter 25

EVALUATING
RESEARCH REPORTS

A. Matching Exercises

Match each of the questions in Set B with the research decision being evaluated, as listed in Set A. Indicate the letter corresponding to your response next to each of the statements in Set B.

SET A
a. Evaluating the research design decisions
b. Evaluating the population and sampling plan
c. Evaluating the data collection procedures
d. Evaluating the analytic decisions

SET B   **RESPONSE**

1. Were there a sufficient number of subjects?   _____

2. Was there evidence of adequate reliability and validity? _____

3. Would a more limited specification have controlled some
   extraneous variables not covered by the research design? _____

4. Would nonparametric tests have been more appropriate?   _____

5. Were respondents assured anonymity or confidentiality?   _____

6. Were threats to internal validity adequately controlled? _____

7. Were the statistical tests appropriate, given the level of measurement of the variables?   _____

8. Were response-set biases minimized?   _____

Polit DF, Hungler BP: STUDY GUIDE FOR NURSING RESEARCH:
PRINCIPLES AND METHODS, 5th ed. © 1995 J.B. Lippincott Company.

9. Was the comparison group equivalent to the experimental group? _____

10. Should the data have been collected prospectively? _____

11. Were triangulation procedures used as a method of validation? _____

12. Were constant comparison procedures appropriately used to refine relevant categories? _____

13. Did the researcher stay in the field long enough to gain an emic perspective? _____

14. Were informants asked to comment on the emerging themes? _____

B. Completion Exercises

Write the words or phrases that correctly complete the sentences below.

1. The research process involves numerous methodological _____ _____, each of which could affect the quality of the study.

2. A good critique should identify both _____ and _____ in a scientific study.

3. An evaluation of the relevance of a study to some aspect of the nursing profession involves critiquing the _____ _____ dimension of a research study.

4. An evaluation of the researcher's plan to avoid self-selection biases involves critiquing the _____ _____ dimension of a research study.

5. An evaluation of the way in which human subjects were treated involves critiquing the _____ _____ dimension of a research study.

6. An evaluation of the sense the researcher tried to make of the results involves critiquing the _____ _____ dimension of the research study.

7. An evaluation of the objectivity of the research report involves critiquing the

_____

_____ dimension of the research study.

C. Study Questions

1. Define the following terms. Compare your definitions with the definitions in Chapter 25 or in the glossary.

    a. Critique: _____

    _____

    _____

    b. Research decisions: _____

    _____

    _____

    c. Methodological dimension: _____

    _____

    _____

2. Read and critique one or more of the following articles (or other articles in the nursing research literature), and apply the questions in Chapter 25 of the text to the article. Prepare two to three pages of "bullet points" that indicate the major strengths and weaknesses of the study.

    • Allan, J. D., Mayo, K., & Michel, Y. (1993). Body size values of white and black women. *Research in Nursing and Health, 16,* 323–333.
    • Baker, C. F., Garvin, B. J., Kennedy, C. W., & Polivka, B. J. (1993). The effect of environmental sound and communication on CCU patients' heart rate and blood pressure. *Research in Nursing and Health, 16,* 415–421.
    • Fuller, B. F., Roberts, J. E., & McKay, S. (1993). Acoustical analysis of maternal sounds during the second stage of labor. *Applied Nursing Research, 6,* 8–12.
    • Griffin, C., Dougherty, M. C., & Yarandi, H. (1994). Pelvic muscles during rest: Responses to pelvic muscle exercise. *Nursing Research, 43,* 164–167.
    • Herth, K. A. (1993). Humor and the older adult. *Applied Nursing Research, 6,* 146–153.
    • Kearney, M. H., Murphy, S., & Rosenbaum, M. (1994). Learning by losing: Sex and fertility on crack cocaine. *Qualitative Nursing Research, 4,* 142–162.

- Laschinger, H. K. S., & Goldenberg, D. (1993). Attitudes of practicing nurses as predictors of intended care behavior with persons who are HIV positive. *Research in Nursing and Health, 16,* 441–450.
- Medley, F., Stechmiller, J., & Field, A. (1993). Complications of enteral nutrition in hospitalized patients with artificial airways. *Clinical Nursing Research, 2,* 212–223.
- Millette, B. E. (1993). Client advocacy and the moral orientation of nurses. *Western Journal of Nursing Research, 15,* 607–618.
- Tombes, M. B., & Gallucci, B. (1993). The effects of hydrogen peroxide rinses on the normal oral mucosa. *Nursing Research, 42,* 332–337.

3. Read the following study and identify its major strengths and limitations: Gilbert, D. A. (1993). Reciprocity of involvement activities in client-nurse interactions. *Western Journal of Nursing Research, 15,* 674–687.

   Now, read Weiss' commentary of Gilbert's study that immediately follows the report (pages 687–688). Do any of your comments overlap with those of Weiss? Do you agree or disagree with Weiss' comments?

D. Application Exercises

At the end of this *Study Guide,* in Part VII, are two actual research reports, one for a qualitative study and the other for a quantitative study. Read one or both of these reports, and prepare a three- to five-page critique summarizing the major strengths and weaknesses of the study.

E. Special Projects

1. Prepare a list of the 10 most important questions that would need to be addressed in a critique of the methodological dimensions of a qualitative study.

2. Rewrite Nelson's report in Chapter 13 of Polit and Hungler's (1993) textbook, *Essentials in Nursing Research,* pages 388–400, using some of the suggestions from the critique.

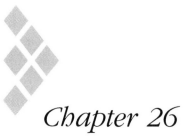

Chapter 26

UTILIZATION OF NURSING RESEARCH

A. Matching Exercises

Match each of the strategies from Set B with one of the roles indicated in Set A. Indicate the letter corresponding to your response next to each of the strategies in Set B.

SET A

a. Nursing researchers
b. Nursing faculty and educators
c. Practicing nurses and nursing students
d. Nursing administrators

SET B   **RESPONSE**

1. Become involved in journal club   _____
2. Perform replications   _____
3. Prepare integrative reviews of research literature   _____
4. Offer resources for utilization projects   _____
5. Disseminate findings   _____
6. Specify clinical implications of findings   _____
7. Read research reports critically   _____
8. Foster intellectual curiosity in the work environment   _____
9. Provide a forum for communication between clinicians and
   researchers   _____
10. Expect evidence that a procedure is effective   _____

Polit DF, Hungler BP: STUDY GUIDE FOR NURSING RESEARCH:
PRINCIPLES AND METHODS, 5th ed. © 1995 J.B. Lippincott Company.

B. Completion Exercises

Write the words or phrases that correctly complete the sentences below.

1. _____

   _____ refers to the use of some aspect of a scientific investigation in an application unrelated to the original research.

2. There is considerable concern about the _____ _____ between knowledge production and knowledge utilization.

3. The most well-known nursing research utilization project, conducted in Michigan, is the _____ _____ Project.

4. An early regional collaborative utilization project was the _____ _____ Project.

5. For research results to be believable, study findings must be _____ _____ in several different settings.

6. The three broad classes of criteria for research utilization are _____ _____, clinical relevance, and scientific merit.

7. The issue of _____ _____ concerns whether it makes sense to implement an innovation in a new practice setting.

8. A cost/benefit assessment should consider not only the net cost or gain of implementing an innovation but also _____ _____.

C. Study Questions

1. Define the following terms. Compare your definition with the definition in Chapter 26 of the textbook or in the glossary.

   a. Instrumental utilization: _____

   _____

   _____

   b. Conceptual utilization: _____

   _____

   _____

   c. Knowledge creep: _____

   _____

   _____

   d. Decision accretion: _____

   _____

   _____

   e. Awareness stage of adoption: _____

   _____

   _____

   f. Persuasion state of adoption: _____

   _____

   _____

   g. Scientific merit: _____

   _____

   _____

   h. Cost/benefit ratio: _____

   _____

   _____

2. Prepare an example of a research question that could be posed to improve nursing care in the five phases of the nursing process.

   a. Assessment phase
   b. Diagnosis phase

    c. Planning phase

    d. Intervention phase

    e. Evaluation phase

3. Think about a nursing procedure about which you have been instructed. What is the basis for this procedure? Determine whether the procedure is based on scientific evidence indicating that the procedure is effective. If it is not based on scientific evidence, on what is it based, and why do you think scientific evidence was not used?

4. Identify the factors in your own setting that you think facilitate or inhibit research utilization (or, in an educational setting, the factors that promote or inhibit a climate in which research utilization is valued.)

5. Read either Brett's (1987) article regarding the adoption of 14 nursing innovations ("Use of nursing practice research findings," *Nursing Research, 36,* pp. 344–349) or the more recent (1990) replication study based on the same 14 innovations by Coyle and Sokop ("Innovation adoption behavior among nurses," *Nursing Research, 39,* pp. 176–180). For each of the 14 innovations, indicate whether you are aware of the findings, persuaded that the findings should be used, use the findings sometimes in a clinical situation, or use the findings always in a clinical situation.

    1. _____

    2. _____

    3. _____

    4. _____

    5. _____

    6. _____

    7. _____

    8. _____

    9. _____

  10. _____

  11. _____

  12. _____

  13. _____

  14. _____

6. With regard to the 14 innovations selected in Brett's study (see Exercise 5 above), select an innovation or finding of which you (or most class members) were unaware. Go to the original source, and read the research report. Perform a

critique of the study, indicating in particular why you think there may have been barriers to having the innovation implemented in a local setting.

D. *Application Exercise*

Below are several suggested research articles. Read one or more of these articles, paying special attention to the Conclusions/Implications section of the report. Evaluate the extent to which you believe the researchers' discussion would facilitate the utilization of the study findings within clinical settings. If possible, suggest some clinical implications that the researchers did not discuss, or discuss the implications in terms of nursing education.

- Brown, S. J. (1994). Communication strategies used by an expert nurse. *Clinical Nursing Research, 3,* 43–56.
- Giuffre, M., Heidenreich, T., & Pruitt, L. (1994). Rewarming cardiac surgery patients: Radiant heat versus forced warm air. *Nursing Research, 43,* 174–178.
- Keeling, A. W., Knight, E., Taylor, V., & Nordt, L. (1994). Postcardiac catheterization time-in-bed study: Enhancing patient comfort through nursing research. *Applied Nursing Research, 7,* 14–17.
- Metheny, N., Reed, L., Wiersema, L., McSweeney, M., Wehrle, M. A., & Clark, J. (1993). Effectiveness of pH measurements in predicting feeding tube placement: An update. *Nursing Research, 42,* 324–331.
- Tombes, M. B., & Gallucci, B. (1993). The effects of hydrogen peroxide rinses on the normal oral mucosa. *Nursing Research, 42,* 332–337.

E. *Special Project*

1. Select a study from the nursing research literature. Using the utilization criteria indicated in Box 26-2 of the textbook, assess the potential for utilizing the study results in a clinical practice setting. If the study meets the three major classes of criteria for utilization, develop a utilization plan.
2. Read the reports on the utilization project conducted under the auspices of the Association of Women's Health, Obstetric, and Neonatal Nurses (AWHONN):

   - Meier, P. P. (1994). Transition of the preterm infant to an open crib: Process of the project group. *Journal of Obstetric, Gynecologic, and Neonatal Nursing, 23,* 321–326.
   - Medoff-Cooper, B. (1994). Transition of the preterm infant to an open crib. *Journal of Obstetric, Gynecologic, and Neonatal Nursing, 23,* 329–335.
   - Gelhar, D. K., Miserendino, C. A., O'Sullivan, P. L., & Vessey, J. A. (1994). Research from the research utilization project: Environmental temperatures. *Journal of Obstetric, Gynecologic, and Neonatal Nursing, 23,* 341–344.

   Evaluate the efficacy of this utilization project.

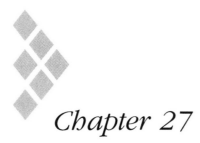

Chapter 27

WRITING A RESEARCH PROPOSAL

A. Matching Exercises

Match each statement designating a section of a National Institutes of Health grant application from Set B with one (or more) of the phrases listed in Set A. Indicate the letter(s) corresponding to your response next to each of the statements in Set B.

SET A
a. Specific Aims section
b. Background and Significance section
c. Preliminary Studies section
d. Research Design and Methods section
e. None of these sections

SET B   RESPONSE

1. Includes the budget   _____

2. Includes a review of previous research   _____

3. Includes a summary of the study objectives   _____

4. Is restricted to three pages   _____

5. Includes a description of the proposed sample   _____

6. Has no explicit page limitations   _____

7. Allows the investigators to elaborate their research qualifications   _____

8. Includes rationales for methodological decisions   _____

9. Has a recommended page limitation of one page   _____

10. May include the work plan   _____
11. Includes biographic sketches   _____
12. Has a recommended page limitation of two to three pages   _____

B. Completion Exercises

Write the words or phrases that correctly complete the sentences below.

1. Proposals often begin with a brief synopsis or _____

   _____ of the proposed research.

2. Objectives stated in the form of _____

   _____ to be tested are generally preferred.

3. The _____

   _____ describes the plan and schedule according to which project tasks would

   be accomplished.

4. The _____

   _____ translates the project activities into monetary terms.

5. A funding agency often publicizes the _____

   _____ that will be used in making evaluative

   decisions about submitted proposals.

6. The person who plays the lead role on a research project is often referred to as

   the _____

   _____ .

7. Applications for research funds through the National Institutes of Health (NIH)

   that are not approved for funding are either _____

   _____ or _____ .

8. The first part of the dual review system within NIH involves a _____

   _____ .

9. Applications to the Public Health Service that are approved for funding are all

   assigned a _____

   _____ .

10. Written critiques of grant applications through the NIH are provided on the

    _____

    _____ .

11. The two major types of federal disbursements are _____

    _____ and _____ .

12. RFP is an acronym for _____

    _____ .

C. Study Questions

1. Define the following terms. Compare your definition with the definition in Chapter 27 of the textbook or in the glossary.

   a. Proposal: _____

      _____

      _____

   b. Work plan: _____

      _____

      _____

   c. Gantt chart: _____

      _____

      _____

   d. Application kit: _____

      _____

      _____

   e. R01 grant: _____

      _____

      _____

   f. AREA award: _____

      _____

      _____

g. FIRST award: _____

_____

_____

h. Priority rating or score: _____

_____

_____

i. Study Section: _____

_____

_____

j. Front matter: _____

_____

_____

k. RFA: _____

_____

_____

l. Grant: _____

_____

_____

m. Contract: _____

_____

_____

2. Chapter 27 of the text described several major sections of Public Health Service grant applications. In which sections would the following statements ordinarily be found?

a. The third task, the screening of volunteers for eligibility and the assignment of subjects to experimental and control groups, will be accomplished in the fourth week of the project and will require 5 person-days of effort. _____

_____

_____

b. The primary hypothesis is that paraplegics who receive pool therapy will perform better on tests of muscle strength than those who receive other types of exercise. _____

_____

_____

c. Dr. Letzeiser, who will direct the proposed research, has recently completed a 3-year longitudinal study of the coping mechanisms of parents with a Down syndrome infant. _____

_____

d. The major threat to the internal validity of the proposed study is selection bias, which will be dealt with through the careful selection of comparison subjects and through statistical adjustment of preexisting differences. _____

_____

_____

e. All subjects will be asked to sign informed consent forms. _____

_____

_____

f. The proposed research will have the potential of restructuring the delivery of health care in rural areas. _____

_____

_____

D. Application Exercises

1. Below is a Specific Aims section from a grant application that was funded by the U.S. Office of Adolescent Pregnancy Programs.* This application is also referred to in Chapter 27 of the text.

*D. Polit, "Parenting among low-income teenage mothers," awarded to Humanalysis, Inc., 1985. Reprinted with permission of Humanalysis, Inc.

SPECIFIC AIMS

Substantial percentages of children in our society are born to young women who are teenagers. Despite the growth of interest in the "epidemic" of teenage pregnancy, relatively little attention has been paid to the parenting styles and behaviors of young mothers or to the development of their children, particularly in well-designed, longitudinal research.

The proposed research will use a combined observational/interview approach to collect information about the parental styles and attitudes, the family and home environment, and children's development in a sample of about 300 low-income young women who first became pregnant when they were 17 or younger, and whose oldest child is now about 5 years of age. Three rounds of interviews with these mothers have already been completed, in which extensive information about their backgrounds, economic circumstances, social support networks, household structure, psychological characteristics, and use of formal services (including parenting education) was gathered. The baseline interviews with these women, conducted either during their pregnancy or shortly after delivery, also measured parenting knowledge and perceived competence in parenting skills. The women in the sample reside in six geographically dispersed communities (Bedford-Stuyvesant, NY; Harlem, NY; Phoenix, AZ; San Antonio, TX; Riverside, CA; and Fresno, CA) and represent an ethnic mix of black, Hispanic, and white young mothers.

The longitudinal nature of this research will make it possible to test a comprehensive model of the effects of maternal age on several parenting and child development outcomes. The availability of extensive background information will also permit background influences (such as pre-delivery family structure and financial circumstances, early school experiences, educational aspirations, self-esteem, and family size expectations) to be controlled, yielding a more sensitive test of the hypothesized effects. In brief, the proposed research will examine the extent to which a teen mother's parenting knowledge is influenced by her age at first birth and her exposure to parenting education classes, net of other factors. Parenting behaviors (such as warmth, punitiveness, and stimulation of the child's learning) are hypothesized to be influenced by three major factors: characteristics of the mother (including her parenting knowledge), characteristics of the child, and contextual factors such as stress and social support. Finally, the model predicts that child development outcomes (including cognitive development, social/behavioral adjustment, and physical health) are a function of parenting behaviors and the home environment, as well as characteristics of the child.

Review and critique this section of the grant application. To assist you in your critique, here are some guiding questions:

a. Is the presentation sufficiently specific? Does the author make overly general statements about what the research will accomplish?

b. Is the presentation clear and succinct? Is it direct and to the point?

c. Does the presentation sound convincing and authoritative? Does the researcher seem knowledgeable about the substantive issues?

d. Do the objectives sound manageable? That is, does it appear that the researcher will actually be able to accomplish her objectives, or is the scope of her objectives overly broad?

2. A nurse researcher wanted to study student attrition among minority nursing school students.† She proposed a critical incidents study of the experiences leading to minority students' decisions to drop out of their nursing programs. The study was to involve interviews with 150 minority dropouts in three states. Below is a tentative budget for such a project.

BUDGET-MINORITY ATTRITION STUDY

Personnel

Rodgers (Principal Investigator)	40 wks @ 800/wk	$32,000
Campbell (Interviewer)	10 wks @ 400/wk	4,000
Wolfe (Interviewer)	10 wks @ 400/wk	4,000
Kulka (Research Assistant)	16 wks @ 275/wk	4,400
Cherlin (Admin. Assistant)	26 wks @ 325/wk	8,450
		$52,850
+ Fringe Benefits (25%)		13,213
TOTAL PERSONNEL		$66,063

Nonpersonnel

Supplies 50/mo. × 12 mos.	$ 600
Xeroxing 50/mo. × 12 mos.	600
Printing Instruments	500
Data entry 300 records × .50/record	150
Travel 3000 miles × 0.25/mile	750
Consultants 10 days @ 250/day	2,500
TOTAL NONPERSONNEL	$ 5,100
TOTAL DIRECT COSTS	**$71,163**

Review and comment on this budget in terms of the following:

a. The inclusion of all relevant budget categories for the proposed study.

b. Your perceptions of whether any given category is over- or underbudgeted.

E. Special Projects

1. Prepare a one-page Special Aims section for a research project you would like to conduct.

2. Identify at least one federal agency and two foundations that might be appropriate for sending a research proposal for a project in which you are interested.

---

†This example is fictitious.

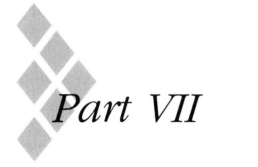

Part VII

RESEARCH
REPORTS

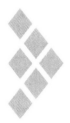

EFFECTS OF A PROCEDURAL/BELIEF INTERVENTION ON BREAST SELF-EXAMINATION PERFORMANCE

Victoria Champion
Catherine Scott

The purpose of this study was to test the effect of a theoretically based nurse-delivered intervention on BSE behavior. A 2 × 2 prospective, randomized, factorial design yielded four groups: control, belief intervention, procedural intervention, and procedural/belief intervention. A total of 301 women were randomly selected from a target population. One year following intervention, significant differences in self-reported proficiency, observer-rated proficiency, and sensitivity (lump detection) were found between the Procedural and Control Group and the Procedural/Belief and Control Group. Significant increases were found on observer-rated proficiency and sensitivity for the Procedural/Belief Group when compared to the Belief Group. In addition, a significant increase was found in the Procedural/Belief Group on nodule detection, when compared to the Procedural Group alone. © 1993 John Wiley & Sons, Inc.

Victoria Champion, DNS, is a professor and Associate Dean for Research, School of Nursing, Indiana University. Catherine Scott, BSN, is a doctoral student in nursing at Indiana University.

This study was supported by NCNR Grant No. NR01843-03.

Champion, V., & Scott, C. (1993). Effects of a procedural/belief intervention on breast self-examination performance. *Research in Nursing and Health, 16,* 163–170. Reprinted with permission.

Requests for reprints can be addressed to Dr. Victoria Champion, Indiana University, School of Nursing, 1111 Middle Drive, Indianapolis, IN 46202-5107.

The incidence of breast cancer continues to rise. The most recent estimates indicate that 186,000 new breast cancers will be detected in the United States in 1992 (Boring, Squires, & Tong, 1992). The best way to lower mortality rates from breast cancer is early diagnosis; 91% of patients with breast cancer discovered at Stage I will be alive in 5 years as opposed to 18% of those whose tumors have advanced to Stage IV (American Cancer Society, 1991).

Breast self-examination (BSE) remains a recommended supplement to mammography and clinical breast examination for enhancing early detection of breast cancers. A number of investigators have found a mortality or stage benefit for women practicing BSE (Foster & Constanza, 1984; Huguley & Brown, 1981; Huguley, Brown, Greenberg, & Clark, 1988; Koroltchouck, Stanley & Stjernsward, 1990; Locker et al., 1989). The purpose of this study was to test selected belief and/or procedural interventions to increase self-reported BSE frequency and proficiency, observer-rated proficiency and sensitivity using a probability sample of women 35 years of age and older.

Many approaches have been used to examine the effects of interventions on increasing BSE frequency, proficiency and, in a few cases, sensitivity. Approaches have varied from handing out pamphlets to prospective randomized trials that include multiple interventions. Some investigators have measured only frequency as the outcome variable (Edgar & Shamian, 1987; Nettles-Carlson, Field, Friedman, & Smith, 1988); others have included proficiency and lump detection (Baines & To, 1990; Fletcher et al., 1990; Worden et al., 1990).

The Health Belief Model (HBM) has influenced research related to BSE behavior. According to the HBM, individuals who have a certain constellation of beliefs will be more likely to carry out a behavior (Rosenstock, 1966). Theoretically, beliefs associated with BSE would be perceived susceptibility to breast cancer, perceived seriousness of breast cancer, perceived benefits of BSE, and few perceived barriers to BSE. It follows, then, that interventions could be aimed at developing the optimal set of beliefs set forth by the HBM that would result in increased BSE behavior.

Health Belief Model (HBM) variables of perceived susceptibility to and seriousness of breast cancer, as well as perceived benefits of and barriers to BSE, have been related to BSE behavior (Champion, 1990; Lashley, 1987; Ronis & Kaiser, 1989; Rutledge, 1987). Worden, Constanza, Foster, Lang, and Tidd (1983) addressed beliefs about susceptibility and benefits using slide/tape presentations with women's groups. Six months after intervention BSE frequency had increased from 40 to 71%. Several other investigators have tested strategies aimed at changing beliefs to be theoretically consistent with the desired behavior (Baker, 1989; Calnan & Rutter, 1986; Carter, Feldman, Tierfer, & Hausdorff, 1985; Mahloch et al., 1990; Nettles-Carlson et al., 1988; Paskett et al., 1990; Worden et al., 1990). Baker (1989) found that a teaching strategy that included work with the HBM variables of susceptibility, seriousness, benefits, and barriers resulted in increased frequency and proficiency in a group of 194 older women 3 months after the intervention. Worden et al., (1990) found on a second year follow-up that women who had barriers addressed had higher scores for sensitivity, frequency, and proficiency than women who had not had this intervention.

Although there have been attempts to incorporate HBM variables into BSE interventions, more work is needed. Many investigators have used only frequency as an outcome measure without adequate attention to proficiency. Even when proficiency was considered, self-reported proficiency, with its potential for social desirability bias, was the primary measurement modality. In addition, short time intervals of 3 to 6 months without measures of long-term change often have been used. Finally, past approaches have not individualized teaching by evaluating pretest scores and addressing only salient belief variables. It is necessary to determine if individualized interventions to alter beliefs added to routine BSE teaching will increase BSE outcome behaviors over and above normal procedural teaching alone. Finally, we need valid and reliable measures of BSE, including observed proficiency and a measure of sensitivity (lump detection).

The 2 × 2 factorial design used for this study incorporated four groups: (a) control, (b) belief intervention, (c) procedural intervention and, (d) procedural/belief interventions. The HBM variables of perceived susceptibility, seriousness, benefits, barriers, health motivation, and control framed the belief intervention. The procedural intervention consisted of a standardized BSE teaching protocol, *Special Touch,* utilized by the American Cancer Society (American Cancer Society, 1987) that involved return demonstration and feedback. Observed proficiency and a measure of sensitivity (lump detection) were added to the measurements of outcome variables.

Hypotheses

1. There will be significant differences between experimental and control groups in self-reported frequency and proficiency of BSE and in observer-rated proficiency and sensitivity one year following intervention.
2. There will be significant increases in self-reported BSE frequency and proficiency and in observer-rated proficiency and sensitivity one year following intervention in the group receiving both belief and procedural protocols when compared to the groups receiving only one of these interventions.

❖ METHOD

Sample

Random-digit dialing was used to produce a probability sample of women 35 years and older who had not developed breast cancer. Telephone solicitors dialed computer-generated random numbers from a large midwestern metropolitan area and its surrounding counties. If there was not an answer, the number was redialed at least 10 times. When an eligible woman was contacted, the study was explained and the woman asked to participate. Women were randomly assigned to one of four groups and assessed on belief variables. An in-home interview was then conducted at which time the intervention was delivered. Women were interviewed one year following intervention to measure outcome variables.

Thirty-three percent of eligible women who were contacted agreed to participate in a larger longitudinal study (2½ years) and completed a baseline survey. Of the initial 322 women who completed the first two phases of data collection, 94% were available for follow-up one year later ($N = 301$).

Demographic characteristics of the sample population were similar to the general target population. Approximately 90% were white, 8% were black, and the remaining Asian or Indian. The mean age for the sample was 50 years ($SD = 12.15$), with a range from 35 to 88. The mean educational level was 13.7 years ($SD = 2.66$) with a range from 8 to 20. Women were paid $25.00 for each in-home interview.

Intervention

BELIEF INTERVENTION. Women in the Belief and Procedural/Belief Groups who had belief scores at the midpoint or below for susceptibility, seriousness, benefits, and health motivation or control and midpoint or above for barriers were targeted for interventions. Belief interventions consisted of counseling individuals about their beliefs when they were not theoretically consistent with desired behavior. Pamphlets with appropriate belief messages were used in the intervention and left with the participant. For the susceptibility intervention, a pamphlet was used which described susceptibility factors for breast cancer. The individual's risk factors were also discussed. The seriousness pamphlet included statistics related to death from breast cancer. The benefits intervention explained the benefits of finding a lump early. The barriers pamphlet discussed common barriers women perceive in relation to BSE and offered suggestions to overcome these barriers. Health motivation and control interventions were aimed at increasing each woman's perception of the importance of general health and her personal control over health.

Extensive training and written materials were provided for research assistants. A training film was produced in which role modeling for each intervention was illustrated. In addition, the principal investigator trained the research assistants by watching them demonstrate the intervention and providing corrective feedback.

PROCEDURAL INTERVENTION. A teaching program based on American Cancer Society recommendations for BSE procedure(s) was delivered to women in the Procedural and Procedural/Belief Groups (American Cancer Society, 1987). Registered nurse graduate students were trained and certified by the ACS to deliver the intervention. A breast model (Health Edco, 1992) was used for demonstrating BSE technique and for the return demonstration. Women were instructed to use adequate pressure for lump detection. Lumps were embedded in the model to allow women the experience of feeling a lump.

Measures

Measurement of HBM variables was accomplished by asking subjects to respond to a series of belief statements, with responses on summated 5-point Likert scales from *strongly agree* to *strongly disagree*. The scale included items for susceptibility, seriousness, benefits, barriers, health motivation, and control. The scales were originally developed by Champion (Champion, 1984) and revised extensively for this research project (Champion, in press). A panel of three national experts who had previously worked with the HBM theory assessed each item for content validity. Consensus was obtained before the item was retained.

All belief scales were assessed for criterion and construct validity. Construct validity was assessed by exploratory factor analysis. Criterion validity was assessed by correlating the entire scale and subscales (susceptibility, seriousness, benefits, barriers, health motivation, and control) with the criterion measure of BSE behavior (R^2 = .24, $p \leq$ .001). Scales were tested for internal consistency and test-retest reliabilities. Internal consistency reliabilities were good and ranged from .80 to .93. Test-retest correlations were moderate, ranging from .45 to .70 (see Table 1). A time lag of between 2 to 8 weeks may have decreased test-retest reliabilities. In addition, the problem of testing effects may have lowered reliabilities, a problem addressed by Carmines and Zeller (1979). Extensive validity and reliability analyses were completed and are reported in detail elsewhere (Champion, in press).

FREQUENCY AND PROFICIENCY OF SELF-REPORTS. Women were asked about the total number of times they had done BSE in the last 12 months (frequency) and about their technique (proficiency) using BSE behavior scales. Items assessed positioning of hands, areas of breasts covered, and other proficiency issues addressed by the American Cancer Society (American Cancer Society, 1987). All items were scored so that increasing magnitude indicated better practice. The BSE behavior scale had a Cronbach alpha of .73 and test-retest reliability of .74. Content validity was assessed by consensus of three experts who were BSE trainers. Confirmatory factor analyses established construct validity.

Table 1.   *Statistics for HBM Scales*

SCALE	M	SD	CRONBACH ALPHA	TEST-RETEST CORRELATION	# ITEMS
Susceptibility	2.54	.81	.93	.70	6
Seriousness	3.25	.68	.80	.45	8
Benefits	3.88	.52	.80	.45	6
Barriers	2.02	.60	.88	.65	7
Health motivation	3.78	.59	.83	.67	8
Control	4.04	.55	.80	.46	4

OBSERVATION OF PROFICIENCY. Participants were observed doing BSE on a model and their performance scored by the graduate nurse research assistant. Because some women were not comfortable returning a demonstration on themselves, all women were tested using the model. The observer checklist contained 10 procedural components that are important for BSE and that corresponded to items included in the self-report BSE measurement scale. Items included positioning of hands and breast area covered, as well as the other items listed in the self-report instrument. Participants were given 2 points for each of eight steps that were adequately completed. Participants were given 4 points each for the last two items since these items involved both position and examination of each breast. Partial credit was given when a step was only partially completed. A total of 24 points was possible on the proficiency checklist. An interobserver reliability of .90 was obtained by having four research assistants simultaneously score four different BSE demonstrations and calculating a coefficient based on the ratio of agreements to agreement plus disagreement.

SENSITIVITY. Participants were assessed on how many nodules embedded in a breast model (Health Edco, 1992) they could identify. A total of five nodules were embedded, and 1 point was given for each nodule identified.

Procedure

After being contacted by telephone and agreeing to participate, all subjects were sent the consent form and the initial survey to assess belief variables. The forms were completed and returned by mail (Time 1), after which research assistants scheduled in-home interviews (Time 2). A second in-home interview was conducted one year later (Time 3).

Subjects were randomly assigned to one of four groups prior to the in-home interview. For subjects assigned to Belief and Procedural/Belief Groups, research assistants used the initial survey to assess participants' scores on susceptibility, seriousness, benefits, barriers, health motivation, and control and to plan interventions when beliefs on any of the HBM variables were not consistent with desirable BSE behavior. Since BSE behavior is not considered adequate in the population generally, it was decided that an average or below average score on belief variables was not adequate to stimulate behavior; therefore, individuals who scored at or below the mean were targeted for intervention. In a like manner, barrier scores at or above the mean were addressed.

If a participant in the Belief Group did not need any of the belief interventions, only the data collection interview occurred at the first in-home visit. The Procedure-Only Group received the BSE teaching intervention as recommended by the ACS. If the participant was in the Procedural/Belief Group and did not require any belief intervention, the procedural intervention alone and data collection interview were conducted. The Control Group had an in-home interview in which all variables were again assessed but no intervention delivered. All groups had variables assessed a second time, with all but the Control Group having the assessment interview after the intervention was delivered. The time between Time 1 and Time 2 ranged from 2 to 8 weeks with a mean of about 4 weeks. One year following the initial in-home interview (Time 2), a second in-home interview (Time 3) was conducted for all groups to assess the effect of interventions on outcome variables.

All statistical analyses were done using SPSSx (Nie, 1988). *T* tests were used to test for significant differences between pre- and postintervention beliefs. A priori contrasts with a one-way ANOVA were used to test for differences in outcome measures between groups on measures that were collected only at Time 3. Self-reported BSE frequency and proficiency before and after interventions were assessed with MANOVA for repeated measures using Time 1 data as a covariate. The repeated measures program allows for testing of equality between groups at pretest and uses any variation (even if not significant) in analysis of posttest differences; it also allows for assessment of pre- to posttest differences across groups. In addition, the repeated measures analysis is more robust than a covariance approach, making it a preferable technique.

❖ RESULTS

A total of 147 participants from the Belief and the Procedural/Belief Group were given a belief intervention on at least one HBM variable. The numbers of subjects receiving each intervention were as follows: susceptibility (133), seriousness (135), benefits (111), barriers (125), health motivation (139), and control (106).

Baseline and postintervention measurement for all dependent measures are shown in Table 2. Groups were not significantly different on beliefs prior to intervention. Prior to hypotheses testing, data from the Belief and Procedural/Belief groups were examined by correlated *t* tests (repeated measures) to determine if significant differences in beliefs emerged between pretest (Time 1) and immediately following intervention (Time 2). Belief and Procedural/Belief Groups were included in analysis since these were the only groups that had interventions aimed at changing beliefs. Significant differences in the expected direction emerged for all belief variables except susceptibility: seriousness $t = 6.25$, $p \leq .001$; benefits $t = 7.50$, $p \leq .001$; barriers $t = 4.02$, $p \leq .001$; health motivation $t = 5.85$, $p \leq .001$; and control $t = 4.43$, $p \leq .001$).

An ANOVA indicated no significant differences between Experimental and Control in either frequency or proficiency prior to intervention. Hypothesis 1 predicted significant effects of intervention on self-reported frequency and proficiency, and observer rated proficiency and sensitivity. A repeated measures MANOVA (group × time) was used to test for intervention effects across time. A significant interaction effect between time and group was needed to indicate a true intervention effect. Results indicated a significant increase in frequency across time $F(1,296) = 262.10$, $p \leq .001$. The group effect was also significant $F(3,296) = 3.23$, $p = .023$. The interac-

Table 2.   *Pre/Postintervention Statistics for BSE Measures*

	CONTROL GROUP (N = 78)		BELIEF GROUP (N = 74)		PROCEDURAL GROUP (N = 75)		PROCEDURAL/ BELIEF GROUP (N = 73)	
	M	**SD**	**M**	**SD**	**M**	**SD**	**M**	**SD**
FREQUENCY								
Preintervention	5.40	4.45	5.77	4.38	6.43	4.71	7.16	4.83
Postintervention[a]	9.44	4.05	10.54	3.35	10.40	3.10	11.00	2.51
PROFICIENCY								
Preintervention	23.21	5.16	22.44	5.50	22.80	5.32	23.69	5.36
Postintervention[a]	28.23	5.21	28.15	5.84	31.21	4.34	31.77	4.00
OBSERVATION[a]	11.21	5.19	12.18	5.46	17.15	5.32	17.14	5.36
NODULES[a]	2.46	1.27	2.34	1.09	3.37	1.05	3.80	1.00

[a]Data collected 1 year postintervention.

tion effect, however, was nonsignificant, indicating that group differences at 1 year postintervention were due to the additive effect of pretest and posttest differences.

Self-reported proficiency data also were assessed using MANOVA with repeated measures. There was a significant difference in self-reported proficiency between groups $F(3,274) = 5.03$, $p \leq .002$, and across time, $F(1,274) = 281.62$, $p \leq .001$; the interaction effect also was significant, $F(3,274) = 5.69$, $p \leq .001$. The Procedural Only and Procedural/Belief Group had a greater increase in proficiency over time than those who received an intervention aimed at beliefs alone or no intervention. Planned comparisons indicated the Procedural and Procedural/Belief Groups, but not the Belief Group, were significantly different than the Control Group. Planned comparisons also indicated the Procedural and Procedural/Belief Groups were not significantly different in terms of proficiency.

Hypothesis 1 also stated that there would be a significant difference in observer-rated scores for proficiency and sensitivity between Experimental and Control Groups. Using a priori contrasts, the Control Group demonstrated significantly lower observer-rated proficiency and sensitivity than either the Procedural or the Procedural/Belief Group, but not the Belief Group (see Table 3).

To test hypothesis 2, behavioral outcomes of the Procedural/Belief intervention were compared to those of the Belief and Procedural interventions. A priori contrasts between the Belief and Procedural/Belief Group were significant for both the observer-rated proficiency and sensitivity scores, with the Procedural/Belief group attaining higher proficiency (see Table 3). A priori contrasts between the Procedural Group and Procedural/Belief Group intervention revealed significant differences for sensitivity (see Table 3). The mean sensitivity for the Procedural Group was 3.36 (*SD*

Table 3.   *A Priori Contrasts for Observer-Rated Proficiency and Sensitivity*

	OBSERVER RATED PROFICIENCY t VALUE (df = 294)	SENSITIVITY t VALUE (df = 295)
Control versus belief	1.02	.68
Control versus procedural	6.24*	5.03*
Control versus procedural/belief	6.18*	7.40*
Procedural versus procedural/belief	.02	2.35*
Belief versus procedural/belief	5.10*	7.98*

$p \leq .01$.

= 1.05) as compared to 3.80 ($SD = .99$) for the Procedural/Belief Group. A limited range (5 lumps) may have precluded finding greater differences.

❖ DISCUSSION

Self-reported retrospective frequency scores for BSE were not significantly different between groups when pretest differences were controlled. There were significant increases in frequency between pre- and postintervention scores, however, even in the Control Group. This finding probably indicates that the effect of being in the study sensitized women to report increased BSE frequency. Individual attention did act to increase reported frequency and this increase was maintained for 1 year. This result may be important considering that maintaining behavior over time has been found to be difficult (Mayer et al., 1987).

Self-reported proficiency scores illustrate a different pattern. Scores for the Procedural and Procedural/Belief Groups increased more over time than scores for the Control or Belief Groups, indicating an effect from the Procedural and Procedural/Belief interventions. It is also obvious that since frequency differences between groups were nonsignificant when proficiency differences were significant, that frequency alone is not an adequate measure of BSE behavior, thus calling into question reports of studies that address only frequency (Edgar & Shamian, 1987; Nettles-Carlson et al., 1988).

Demonstrations of BSE on models were not done on pretest to partially control for the sensitizing effect of demonstrating the procedure. In addition, since this was a randomized design, groups could be assumed equal on these measures. Nurse-rated proficiency 1 year after intervention was higher in the groups that had received training in the procedure, confirming the usefulness of that intervention. Observer-rated proficiency is probably a more valid indicator of actual technique than are self-report measures since it avoids the problem of self-report bias.

The most important findings are the significant differences that emerged in terms of sensitivity. Both the Procedural Group and the Procedural/Belief Groups were significantly different from the Control or Belief Groups. In addition, the Procedural/Belief Group was significantly different than the group receiving only procedural instruction. Having a theoretically consistent set of beliefs may increase the desire for learning which results in the procedural intervention being more effective. This finding is especially important in light of the need for research with better outcome measures (O'Malley & Fletcher, 1987). This finding also is consistent with Worden et al. (1990), who found that a group in which barriers were assessed had increased sensitivity (lump detection). The possibility must be acknowledged, however, that detection of lumps in a synthetic model would not translate to actual lump detection. It also is difficult to assess the clinical significance of this finding. In addition, false positive lump identification was not measured in this study. It would be impossible, however, to design a study using lump detection in a human as the outcome measure without conducting an extremely large longitudinal study that would extend for years. This study did incorporate the most logical analogue to lump detection in women (lump detection in a synthetic model) an improvement over other studies (Baker, 1989; Grady, 1988; Nettles-Carlson, et al., 1988).

Because this study took place in the participant's home, the results cannot be generalized to clinic settings. There is no reason to think, however, that results would be different in a clinic, and it is even possible that individualized interventions would be more effective when delivered in a medical or health care setting. Although group differences in postintervention self-reported frequency were not found, frequency increases over time were significant for all groups. The effect of interaction with a nurse may have acted as an intervention even for the Control Group. Further research with a no-contact control group may help clarify this finding.

It is encouraging that a high percentage of women (94%) remained in the study after initial intervention. The somewhat low proportion of subjects who initially agreed to participate (33%) does limit generalization. However, refusal to participate was often attributed to reluctance to commit to a 2½ year study and, therefore, it is not surprising that the refusal rate for this study was higher than the rates for cross-sectional studies. It also must be acknowledged that, although approximately 95% of women in the target population had a telephone, results cannot be generalized to those without phones. Generalizability is also limited because participants were relatively well educated and may have been more interested in or motivated to learn about BSE than those who refused. This limitation, however, is common in research with volunteer subjects.

In conclusion, preliminary results indicate that nursing interventions may increase BSE frequency and proficiency over time. Personal contact emphasizing BSE may be all that is needed to increase frequency; however, proficiency was dependent upon a standardized teaching Procedure and/or Procedural/Belief intervention. The lack of difference between Procedural and Procedural/Belief Groups on some outcome measures may have been due in part to the fact that the teaching intervention (the American Cancer Society protocol) also included emphasis on decreasing barriers and increasing control over health, as well as information about susceptibility. Follow-up over longer periods is needed to provide information on long-term effects.

These preliminary findings indicate a statistically significant additive effect for sensitivity when belief interventions are added to procedural teaching. If this is confirmed in subsequent studies, the cost effectiveness of this additional step in teaching BSE should be examined. In addition, targeted and individualized interventions should be compared to a standardized format in which all women receive the same belief intervention regardless of individualized differences.

References

American Cancer Society. (1987). *Special touch facilitators guide,* Atlanta: Author.

American Cancer Society. (1991). *Cancer facts & figures—1991,* Atlanta: Author.

Baines, C. J., & To, T. (1990). Changes in breast self-examination behavior achieved by 89,835 participants in the Canadian National Breast Screening Study. *Cancer, 66,* 570–576.

Baker, J. A. (1989). Breast self-examination and the older woman: Field testing an educational approach. *The Gerontologist, 29,* 405–407.

Boring, M. S., Squires, T., & Tong, T. (1991). Cancer statistics, 1992. *CA—A Cancer Journal for Clinicians, 42*(1), 19–38.

Calnan, M., & Rutter, D. R. (1986). Do health beliefs predict health behaviour? An analysis of breast self-examination. *Social Science & Medicine, 22,* 673–678.

Carmines, E., & Zeller, P. (1979). *Reliability and validity assessment.* Newbury Park, CA: Sage.

Carter, A. C., Feldman, J. G., Tierfer, L., & Hausdorff, J. K. (1985). Methods of motivating the practice of breast self-examination: A randomized trial. *Preventive Medicine, 14,* 555–572.

Champion, V. L. (1984). Instrument development for health belief model constructs. *Advances in Nursing, Science, 6*(3), 73–85.

Champion, V. L. (1990). Breast self-examination in women 35 and older: A prospective study. *Journal of Behavioral Medicine, 13,* 523–528.

Champion, V. L. (in press). Refinement of instruments to measure Health Belief Model constructs. *Nursing Research.*

Edgar, L., & Shamian, J. (1987). Promoting healthy behaviours: The nurse as a teacher of breast self-examination. *HYGIE, 6*(2), 37–41.

Fletcher, S. W., O'Malley, M. S., Earp, J. A. L., Morgan, T. M., Lin, S., & Degnan, D. (1990). How best to teach women breast self-examination. A randomized controlled trial. *Annals of Internal Medicine, 112,* 772–779.

Foster, R. S., & Constanza, M. C. (1984). Breast self-examination practices and breast cancer survival. *Cancer, 53,* 999–1005.

Grady, K. E. (1988). Older women and the practice of breast self-examination. *Psychology of Women Quarterly, 12,* 473–487.

Health Edco. (1992). *Educational products catalog.* Waco, TX.

Huguley, C. M., & Brown, R. L. (1981). The value of breast self-examination. *Cancer, 47,* 989–995.

Huguley, C., Brown, R., Greenberg, R., & Clark, S. (1988). Breast self-examination and survival from breast cancer. *Cancer, 62,* 1389–1396.

Koroltchouk, V., Stanley, K., & Stjernsward, J. (1990). The control of breast cancer. A World Health Organization perspective. *Cancer, 65,* 2803–2810.

Lashley, M. E. (1987). Predictors of breast self-examination practice among elderly women. *Advances in Nursing Science, 9*(4), 25–34.

Locker, A., Caseldine, J., Mitchell, A., Blamey, R., Roebuck, E., & Elston, C. (1989). Results from a seven-year programme of breast self-examination in 89,010 women. *British Journal of Cancer, 60,* 401–405.

Mahloch, J., Paskett, E., Henderson, M., Grizzle, J., Ross-Price, M., & Thompson, R. S. (1990). An evaluation of BSE frequency and quality and their relationship to breast lump detection. *Progress in Clinical & Biological Research, 339,* 269–280.

Mayer, J. A., Dubbert, P. M., Scott, R. R., Dawson, B. L., Ekstrand, M. L., & Fondren, T. G. (1987). Breast self-examination: The effects of personalized prompts on practice frequency. *Behavior Therapy, 2,* 135–146.

Nettles-Carlson, B., Field, M. L., Friedman, B. J., & Smith, L. S. (1988). Effectiveness of teaching breast self-examination during office visits. *Research in Nursing & Health, 11,* 41–50.

Nie, N. H. (1988). *SPSSx user's guide.* New York: McGraw-Hill.

O'Malley, M. S., & Fletcher, S. W. (1987). Screening for breast cancer with breast self-examination. *Journal of the American Medical Association, 257,* 2197–2203.

Paskett, E. D., White, E., Urban, N., Gey, G. O., Hornecker, J., Meadows, S., & Sifferman, F. R. (1990). Implementation and evaluation of a worksite breast self-examination training program. *Progress in Clinical & Biological Research, 339,* 281–302.

Ronis, D. L., & Kaiser, M. K. (1989). Correlates of breast self-examination in a sample of college women: Analyses of linear structural relations. *Journal of Applied Social Psychology, 19,* 1068–1084.

Rosenstock, I. M. (1966). Why people use health services. *Milbank Memorial Fund Quarterly, 44,* 94–121.

Rutledge, D. M. (1987). Factors related to women's practice of breast self-examination. *Nursing Research, 36,* 117–121.

Worden, J. K., Constanza, M. C., Foster, R. S., Lang, S. P., & Tidd, C. A. (1983). Content and context in health education: Persuading women to perform breast self-examination. *Preventive Medicine, 12,* 331–339.

Worden, J. K., Solomon, L. J., Flynn, B. S., Constanza, M. C., Foster, R. S., Dorwaldt, A. L., & Weaver, S. O. (1990). A community-wide program in breast self-examination training and maintenance. *Preventive Medicine, 19,* 254–269.

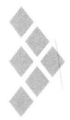

AIDS FAMILY CAREGIVING: TRANSITIONS THROUGH UNCERTAINTY*

Marie Annette Brown
Gail M. Powell-Cope†

The purpose of this study was to describe the experience of AIDS family caregiving. Grounded theory provided the methodological basis for qualitative data generation and analysis. Extensive interviews were conducted with 53 individuals (lovers, spouses, parents of either adults or children with AIDS, siblings, and friends) who were taking care of a person with AIDS at home. Relevant features of the social context of AIDS family caregiving were explored. Findings revealed the basic social psychological problem of Uncertainty, a core category of Transitions Through Uncertainty, and five subcategories: Managing and Being Managed by the Illness; Living With Loss and Dying; Renegotiating the

*Accepted for publication April 8, 1991. Earlier versions of this paper were presented at the 1989 meeting of the Western Institute for Nursing and the 1989 Council of Nurse Researchers meeting. This study was funded in part by a Biomedical Research Support Grant from the University of Washington School of Nursing and the Psi Chapter of Sigma Theta Tau. Although there is a designated first and second author, this article is a result of a collaborative effort between the authors. Both authors contributed equally to the final product. We gratefully acknowledge the generous contribution of time from our study participants. We sincerely appreciate the substantive and methodological assistance provided by Kristen Swanson, PhD, RN, Phil Bereano, PhD, Kimberly Moody, PhC, RN, and Linda Meldman, PhC, RN.

Reprinted here from *Nursing Research* (1991;40[6]:338–345), with permission.

†Marie Annette Brown, PhD, RN, is an associate professor in the School of Nursing, University of Washington, Seattle, WA.

Gail M. Powell-Cope, PhC, RN, is a doctoral candidate in nursing science at the school of Nursing, University of Washington, Seattle, WA.

Relationship; Going Public; and Containing the Spread of HIV. Stages and strategies of each subcategory detailed individuals' responses to the challenges of AIDS family caregiving and elaborated the day-to-day experiences. Uncertainty as a critical challenge for individuals and families facing life-threatening illness is discussed in light of recent research.

The physical and emotional devastation of HIV infection and AIDS produces extraordinary challenges to the health care system. Families and significant others assume heavy responsibilities for care of these individuals and provide the cornerstone of society's response to the AIDS epidemic (Haque, 1989; Wolcott et al., 1986). For example, Raveis and Siegel (1990) found that informal or familial caregivers provided approximately two-thirds of the total assistance required for instrumental activities, transportation, administrative activities, and home medical care for persons with AIDS (PWAs) even though the sample was relatively healthy. Hepburn (1990) emphasized that if family caregivers of PWAs "play a comparable role to informal caregivers of the elderly, they will have significant impact on the overall care and well-being of AIDS patients" (p. 41).

❖ LITERATURE REVIEW

The literature suggests that there are risks to assuming the family caregiver role of an elderly or ill person including physical morbidity (Snyder & Keefe, 1985; Baumgarten, 1989); depression, mental exhaustion, and burnout (Chenoweth & Spencer, 1986; Ekberg, Griffith, & Foxall, 1986; Livingston, 1985); burden, strain (Montgomery, Gonyea, & Hooyman, 1985; Zarit, Todd, & Zarit, 1986); anger, depression, fatigue (Rabins, Mace, & Lucas, 1982; Rabins, Fitting, Eastham, & Fettig, 1990); and uncertainty (Stetz, 1989). Furthermore, parent caregivers of chronically ill children experience changes in the marital relationship, financial constraints, and role alterations (Thomas, 1987). These parent caregivers often become socially isolated as they focus on the ill child, become less available for reciprocal exchange with others, and experience the withdrawal of friends and other family members (Thomas, 1987). It is particularly common that middle-aged caregivers are unable to fulfill their work and family roles adequately (Miller & Montgomery, 1990). In a recent study of informal caregivers of PWAs, alterations in work role performance and economic burden were common, even though the sample consisted of relatively healthy PWAs with few functional disabilities (Raveis & Siegel, 1990). Over one-third of the caregivers had made financial changes in their lives and passed up financial opportunities, and 13% reported somewhat serious financial problems. Most (72%) of those employed reported that their ability to concentrate at work was affected by the patient's illness. A substantial minority (39%) reported arriving at work late or leaving early because the PWA was ill, had to be escorted to a medical appointment, or needed assistance with errands. Twenty-eight percent admitted that in recent months they had to take sick leave, vacation, or personal days because of the PWA's illness (Raveis & Siegel, 1990).

While there may be challenges common for all caregivers, each subgroup of caregivers face unique psychosocial stressors, often related to the characteristics of the care recipient. Issues of communicability, stigma, and multiple and premature losses are common in AIDS family caregiving. The issue of communicability of this "deadly disease" can stimulate fears of contagion and death in loved ones, friends, and coworkers of both the patient and the family caregiver (Ostrow & Gayle, 1986). Coping with AIDS phobia, the stigma associated with homosexuality, bisexuality, or IV drug use, as well as the tremendous demands of caregiving, may become overwhelming for family members (Moffatt, 1986). Schoen (1986) highlighted the additional strain faced by younger caregivers, particularly spouses and lovers, who deal with such a catastrophic, life-threatening illness before reaching half of their life expectancy, and who have not acquired the maturity and perspective that often accompany middle and older age. Caregivers who are HIV positive witness deterioration and death that could forecast their own fate (Shilts, 1987; Edwards, 1988). Lastly, a large proportion of AIDS family caregivers are men, who in American culture usually receive less preparation than women for nurturing roles.

Virtually no information exists about AIDS family caregiving, and much of the general family caregiving research focuses only on caregiving tasks and related effects on the caregiver (Bowers, 1987). The grounded theory method is a particularly important research strategy to address these gaps and serves to "clarify, develop, or redirect research in a content area about which much is already known" (Bowers, 1987, p. 31). Therefore, the purpose of this grounded theory study was to explore and describe the experience of family members who were caring for PWAs at home. The term *family caregiver* employed in this study includes family of origin and family of choice.

❖ METHOD

Sample

Participants were recruited from a variety of AIDS community sources, including clinics, support groups, a caregiver course, volunteer organizations, and a community newspaper. The sample consisted of 53 family caregivers of people with symptomatic HIV infection or AIDS. Approximately one-third (32%) were partners or lovers in gay relationships, 6% were partners or spouses in heterosexual relationships, 43% were friends (9% were former lovers), 13% were parents, 4% were siblings, and 4% were other family of origin. The parents included those of both adult and minor children with HIV/AIDS. Seventy-seven percent lived in the same household with the PWA and 60% of the households also included other individuals such as the caregiver's partner, child, or housemate. Approximately two-thirds (64%) of the family caregivers were male and 36% were female. Approximately two-thirds (68%) were gay or bisexual and 32% were heterosexual. The sample ranged from 22 to 65 years old (*M* = 36). Fifty-seven percent had less than a college degree and 92% were white.

Fifty percent of the caregivers were employed full-time and 19% part-time outside the home. Family incomes (which supported an average of 1.9 persons) were low, with 18% reporting under $10,000, 41% between $10–20,000, 16% $20–30,000, 16% $30–40,000, and 9% over $40,000. In almost half (47%) of the families, the PWA had been diagnosed within the past 12 months. Eighty-four percent of the caregivers knew the PWA prior to the diagnosis of AIDS. The sample contained few ethnic minorities and a large number of caregivers of gay PWAs, thus reflecting the demographics of AIDS in the geographical area where the study was conducted (DSHS & Seattle-King County Health Department, 1991). However, compared to family caregivers of people with other health problems, this sample was younger with a greater proportion of men, fewer spouses, and fewer members from families of origin.

Procedure

After consent was obtained, participants were asked: "What has it been like for you living with and taking care of someone with AIDS?" Relevant probes were used to gain further insight into issues raised. In addition, an interview guide was used to insure consistency of topics across interviews. Interviews were conducted in either one or two sessions, lasted a mean of 4.5 hours, and yielded over 200 hours of interview data. Confidentiality was maintained.

While a triangulation of methods was used to address the study purpose, this paper will include only findings from qualitative analyses. Grounded theory (Glaser & Strauss, 1967; Strauss, 1987) provided the methodological basis for qualitative data generation and analysis. This approach is derived from symbolic interactionism, which focuses on human social and psychological processes as they are grounded in social interaction. The basic tenet of symbolic interactionism is that people construct meanings about phenomenon based on interpretations of interactions they have with one another and with themselves (Blumer, 1969). Therefore, family caregiving is viewed as a socially interactive process that supports the ill person, in this case, the person with HIV infection.

Interviews were tape-recorded and transcribed verbatim. Constant comparative analysis was used as an ongoing technique that included deriving first level codes, or in vivo codes, comparing codes to one another, deriving conceptual categories, and related categories to codes and to other categories. Coding strategies included open coding (unrestricted selection of codes from the search for words or phrases that capture the meaning in the transcripts), axial coding (comparison between codes), and selective coding (utilization of frequently occurring codes to create core categories). Theoretical sampling was accomplished by selecting respondents based on the need to collect more data to examine categories and their relationships, and to ensure representativeness in the category. Theoretical saturation determined the discontinuation of new data collection. Theoretical saturation occurred when information became redundant and a core category was created and linked to subcategories.

Validity and reliability of the data were addressed systematically using the criteria outlined by Sandelowski (1986) and Lincoln and Guba (1985): (a) truth value,

(b) applicability, (c) consistency, and (d) neutrality. Member checks, debriefing by peers, triangulation, prolonged engagement with the data, persistent observation, and reflective journals were techniques used to ensure validity and reliability. During the final phases of analysis, focus groups of study alumni, family caregivers who did not participate in the study, and professionals and community volunteers working in the area of AIDS family caregiving were asked to review and to critique the validity of the substantive theory of AIDS family caregiving. Modifications of the theoretical presentation were made based on feedback from these experts as well as from consensus between the researchers. The categories developed during this study were also validated using literature in the popular press. Examination of Monette's (1988) detailed account of caring for his partner with AIDS revealed evidence of the basic social psychological problem, core category, subcategories, and stages and strategies.

Context and Assumptions

Grounded theory methodology suggests that it is crucial to examine the broader social context of the phenomenon under study. The data from this study represent caregiving that occurred between 1985 and 1988. Caregiving during those years of the AIDS epidemic was inextricably linked to several salient issues: a silent government, a vocal gay community, an unresponsive bureaucracy, inexperienced health care providers, and a frightened, uninformed, and homophobic populace.

Specific aspects of the cultural context can be related to the five subcategories describing caregivers' responses to the challenge of AIDS. For example, complicating the caregivers' attempt to manage the illness was a society that undervalued care provided in the home and traditionally expected women to fulfill that role without compensation or reward. Living with loss and dying was made more difficult by the high value placed on youth and appearance. Pervasive divorce and domestic violence as well as widespread intolerance of nontraditional family compositions undermined the ability to maintain relationships. Because of the societal stigma associated with AIDS and fear of exposure to prejudice, persons with AIDS and caregivers were not encouraged to "go public" with their disease, but instead had to hide the truth.

Moreover, the attempt to contain the spread of HIV was hindered by contradictory messages. On one hand, popular images promoted by the media and embraced by society suggested that romantic sex should ideally be spontaneous and unprotected. While on the other hand, the medical community advised condom use to prevent the transmission of AIDS. Yet despite the information provided by the medical community, their efforts to convince the general public to practice "safe" sex were not adequate.

❖ RESULTS

The substantive theory of AIDS family caregiving developed during this study is outlined in Figure 1. *Uncertainty* was identified as the basic social psychological

Table 1. *Substantive Theory of AIDS Family Caregiving*

BASIC SOCIAL-PSYCHOLOGICAL PROBLEM	CORE CATEGORY	SUBCATEGORIES	STAGES AND STRATEGIES
Uncertainty ⟶	Transitions Through Uncertainty	1. Managing and Being Managed by the Illness	a. Watching and Analyzing b. Doing for c. Coordinating Help
		2. Living with Loss and Dying	a. Facing loss b. Putting the future on hold c. Maximizing the present
		3. Renegotiating the Relationship	a. Modifying give and take b. Coping with dependency c. Minimizing conflicts
		4. Going Public	a. Living with Secrecy b. Asserting oneself c. Balancing risks and benefits
		5. Containing the Spread of HIV	a. Confronting fear and personal vulnerability b. Doing things differently

problem and *Transitions Through Uncertainty* the core category of AIDS family caregiving. In addition to the pervasive sense of uncertainty that characterized the AIDS caregiving transition, the day-to-day experience of uncertainty was best understood in the context of the five caregiving subcategories (Figure 1). These subcategories also highlighted areas of caregivers' lives that were most significant and problematic. Stages and strategies of each subcategory detail caregivers' action-oriented responses to the uncertainties and specific challenges characteristic of each subcategory.

Uncertainty[1]

Uncertainty was identified as the basic social psychological problem in the AIDS caregiving transition. Uncertainty, as conceptualized in this study, is defined as

[1]Although our analysis was conducted without knowledge of Mishel's reconceptualization of the uncertainty in illness theory (1990), the studies contain parallel findings that support an expanded perspective on the acceptance of uncertainty.

the caregiver's inability to predict future events and outcomes and the lack of confidence in making day-to-day decisions about the ill person's care. Uncertainty exerted a profound influence on caregivers' lives and pervaded the entire caregiving experience; it never completely disappeared, but varied in intensity, timing, and content. Even though caregivers reported increasing confidence in their caregiving abilities and increasing ability to predict outcomes over time, uncertainty about some issue always remained. Even after one year of caregiving, one lover expressed some self-doubts:

> So I don't necessarily feel 100% about everything I'm doing, but I have to do it . . . I'm not 100% positive, 100% sure, 100% that it's the right thing to do for Mike . . . It becomes very obscure, blurry, as to whether I'm doing anything right.

Feelings of uncertainty in AIDS family caregiving arose from the perceptual and unpredictable changes accompanying AIDS. The PWA's health or functional ability and the caregivers' emotional responses were often in a constant state of flux. One caregiver emphasized the difficulties in trying to keep abreast of these constant changes:

> It constantly changes. I want to emphasize that. You can't learn what the boundary is, because the boundary of today is not gonna be the boundary of tomorrow. What you've got to learn is how to have an antenna.

Often, study participants spontaneously offered the roller coaster metaphor to describe the constant changes inherent in AIDS caregiving. A roller coaster, with many ups and downs, reflected the relentlessness and the lack of control in AIDS family caregiving. For the most part, caregivers were unable to seek respite from the constant drama of AIDS, and to create a more stable period in the lives. Two different caregivers expressed their feelings about the roller coaster as follows:

> The roller coaster describes the situation in lots of different ways. What's happening to the person's health? What's happening to your feelings? What's happened here today? It's this incredible uncertainty.

> Well, it got to be like an emotional roller coaster, one of these up and down and up and down . . . So it's almost as though you want to tell yourself, well, his condition is stabilized. This stuff doesn't stabilize very long . . .

Uncertainty was problematic for caregivers because of a cultural context that emphasize the need to understand, predict, and/or control events. Caregivers struggled as they faced the contradiction between their expectations about prediction and control and the reality of their personal experiences which were imbued with constant uncertainty. Initially, caregivers expected health care providers to be able to provide them with incontestable information about AIDS and the PWA's course of illness. Caregivers often were frustrated when they turned to health care providers for definitive answers and found that the professionals were themselves equally uncertain. One caregiver expressed his frustration with the inability of the physicians to explain his partner's new and foreboding neurological symptoms:

He's got a malfunction in his brain and no one knows what's going on. The neurosurgeons, and neurologists and doctors at the AIDS clinic . . . No one knows what's happening but it's getting worse.

While some caregivers learned to accept uncertainty over time, others had a stronger need to establish some degree of certainty in their lives. Some caregivers did not want to accept the uncertainty of AIDS caregiving and tried to force certainty where it did not exist. After numerous attempts to exercise control in the face of constant change, many caregivers discovered the fallacy of this imperative and began to accept uncertainty. One caregiver poignantly described his paradoxical reflections about the uncertainty of his lover's mortality:

I like to know what's going to happen in a clear-cut path in a pattern that I can control . . . So my certainty was that I finally decided Mike was going to die. Finally I realized what right do I have to decide the fate of someone else's life? He may not die. I was doing it for my own protection, my own sanity . . . So I opened up that wound, or whatever you call that, and let uncertainty back into my life.

Transitions

A transition is a period of major change in life circumstances accompanied by uncertainty, questioning one's basic assumptions, and reexamining plans for living in the world (Parkes, 1971) which results in the reordering of life activities and a trans-formed self-identity. As a result of prolonged engagement with the data and with the literature, we identified caregiving as a transition to be a critical feature of AIDS family caregiving. Study participants consistently described AIDS caregiving as a significant phase of life as portrayed in the definition above. Many emphasized caregiving as a process that occurred over time or a series of changes. This lover struggled with the effects of dramatic changes in the PWA's health over a short period of time:

You should have talked to me three months ago when he was in the hospital with pneumonia. Life was completely different then: I was a basket case, whirling from the news from AIDS and afraid of death at any moment. Now he's back to work and we seem to be pretending that we are living a normal life.

Others viewed caregiving as a journey or passage, or a path they chose. One man talked about his depth of experience as a caregiver for his lover.

It [caregiving] has been a real path . . . It's a strange time for us right now. It's almost a very spiritual time.

Caregiving may last for only a few months or extend over several years. As in any transition, caregiving demanded time for making meaning of events and experiences as caregivers learned to live and to view their worlds differently. Two partners described the common theme of a life transformed by AIDS caregiving:

Joe was diagnosed a little over one year ago and my life has changed forever . . . things keep happening . . . and I have discovered this past year how much work it is.

He was diagnosed in May with a Kaposi's spot. Up until that time AIDS had never entered our relationship. Nobody ever thought about AIDS . . . It's completely changed our lives in a lot of ways. And where we're at right now is . . . we've almost come full circle now. We've worked out a lot of things this past year, dealing with the disease.

The transition of AIDS caregiving was characterized by both numerous crises and quiescent periods between crises. Common precipitators of crises were usually associated with sudden changes in the PWA's health such as *Pneumocystis* pneumonia, falls, delirium, and acute panic attacks. One caregiver described his frightening experience of finding his lover at home critically ill:

I called him at his apartment and he was very, very sick and he was in a lot of denial. And the reality of it was that he was developing cryptococcal meningitis. He was becoming demented and totally out of it . . He kept dropping the phone and not picking it up. I'd scream into the phone and there'd be no answer . . . finally I said, "I think we've got to go into the hospital." I went to pick him up and he had difficulty buzzing me into the apartment. When I got into the apartment it was a total mess. There was rotting food all over. He didn't know who he was.

The quiescent times between crises were often viewed by caregivers as "good times." Often during these periods caregivers were able to focus more on their own lives, to create a more peaceful existence, and to increase involvement in community and social activities. One lover, who had experienced many crises with the PWA in the past year, now felt a respite from the difficulties and was enjoying a new sense of well-being:

It sounds hard to believe after all these things I've been telling you, but I'm very happy with the way my life is going right now. I have the most wonderful balance in the world, of working at the bakery part-time and being able to live in a very bohemian lifestyle, working in my garden, spending what time I can with Jeff. I am at definitely the most content place in my life than I've been in many, many, many years. I don't think I would do anything different right now.

Managing and Being Managed by the Illness

This subcategory is defined as vigilantly monitoring the mercurial illness of HIV/AIDS and constantly responding to the relentless demands and uncertainties associated with caregiving tasks. The stages and strategies involved in *Managing and Being Managed* include (a) watching and analyzing, (b) doing for,[2] and (c) coordinating help.

Although present in all categories, uncertainty was most dramatic in *Managing and Being Managed* and reflected the recent appearance of AIDS as a new and poorly understood disease. This uncertainty for caregivers was related to questioning how the disease would unfold, monitoring the symptoms, determining the meaning

---

[2]The language and conceptualization of *Doing For* was influenced by Dr. Kristen Swanson's theoretical development of caring published in *Nursing Research* (Vol. 40, No. 3).

of symptoms and illness behavior, deciding about treatment options, evaluating the effectiveness of caregiving strategies, and developing confidence in their ability to care for the PWA.

A common example of uncertainty related to monitoring the illness was the attempt to determine the meaning of the PWA's symptoms. This process was evident in the dilemma called, "Is it him or the disease?" Caregivers often questioned the PWA's behavior by asking, "Is this an emotional response to the disease (e.g. depression) or is this just him?" The uncertainty manifest in this question prompted caregivers to be cautious so that they would not overlook important symptoms. Consequently, they seriously questioned whether each symptom indicated a new manifestation of the disease, such as brain lesion, the beginning of an opportunistic infection, or a milestone suggesting a slow, steady deterioration. In the absence of a physiological explanation, caregivers attempted to resolve the uncertainty by attributing symptoms to the PWA's personality. This form of uncertainty was often very stressful, as expressed by one woman caring for her friend.

> His decision-making skills and abilities could be really impaired and it's important to keep a scope on that in your heads . . . It's like, he's crazy now! You know, it's hard to tell, because like I said, he's a pretty far out there person anyway. It's like, "Do you think he's crazy now? What do you guys think? I don't know . . . Maybe." . . . I mean, he goes out and buys a $300 funeral outfit. Is this crazy behavior?

Being Managed by the Illness resulted from the relentless nature of caregiving activities and seriousness of the PWA's immune system compromised by HIV infection. Despite the numerous activities involved in managing the illness, the feeling of "never being able to do enough" contributed to the perception of being managed. One mother described how the vigilance of monitoring the disease and the uncertainty of the PWA's behavior translated into the feeling of "24 hours a day on call":

> You can't leave him alone too long because you never know how the mind's going to be. You never know things. Like one time I went to sleep and I thought he was in his room and he had checked himself back into the hospital.

For many caregivers, this constant vigilance became a major contributor to the experience of *Being Managed by the Illness*. Overall, the cumulative stresses associated with *Being Managed by the Illness* sometimes resulted in caregiver burnout that seriously affected the individual's quality of life.

Living with Loss and Dying

This subcategory is defined as the process of revising one's plans for living in the world based on the possible or probable death of a loved one. Stages and strategies include: (a) Facing loss, (b) Putting the future on hold, and (c) Maximizing the present.

Three major sources of uncertainty with *Living with Loss and Dying* were described by caregivers: whether to remain hopeful about the PWA's survival, not knowing which illness or opportunistic infection would herald the PWA's death, or not knowing when the death would occur. These uncertainties related to facing loss were very painful for caregivers to contemplate. Yet, death was so commonplace in those with AIDS, and the threat of death so powerful, that most caregivers were unable to deny the reality of a probable death. One man described the uncertainty of his partner's survival during an acute illness:

> The doctor said, "You know I don't know . . ." Well, actually when Matt first went into the hospital he was so sick the doctor said, "I don't know if he'll live through the evening or he'll live for . . ." As the doctor told me, "He might die tonight, he might die in six months." That was the time for him given. And I thought, "Well, hmmmm, this is an interesting situation."

Another man wondered how the dying process of his lover would unfold:

> Sometimes I wonder "Will he, you know, will his immune system just sort of fall apart, and will he have multiple opportunists and die fairly quickly, within a matter of a few months, or will there be a prolonged time of morbidity, lots of time in the hospital, lots of time in which he feels bad and needs emotional support from me and dies?"

Both the long-range and short-term future were constant sources of uncertainty for caregivers. Even plans for the most immediate future—tomorrow, this weekend—were always uncertain because they were contingent on the PWA's strength and symptomology. Living "one day at a time" became an anchor in the lives of many caregivers as they struggled with an uncertain future and focused on the present.

Renegotiating the Relationship

This subcategory is defined as the ongoing process of revising the rules and expectations and striving to reach acceptable balances. Stages and strategies include (a) Modifying give and take, (b) Coping with dependency, and (c) Minimizing conflict. Uncertainty within *Renegotiating the Relationship* focused on questioning one's commitment to caregiving, the rules and expectations of the relationship given the PWA's illness, and appropriate strategies for interpersonal conflict with someone who may die soon.

At the outset of illness or the diagnosis of AIDS, caregivers often faced the fundamental question: "Am I willing to do this?" However, many caregivers did not recall consciously choosing to become a caregiver, and instead naturally assumed the role given the nature of their relationship with the PWA. For some caregivers, the increasing strains and demands associated with caregiving provoked uncertainty about staying in or leaving the relationship. Despite his initial commitment to caregiving, one 24-year-old man questioned whether he could continue caring for his lover and cope with the constant changes in their relationship brought about by AIDS:

Like any other relationship, you have your ups and downs, and sometimes there's more downs than ups . . . maybe it's better for us to . . . you have to decide whether it's healthier to be in a relationship or healthier to not be in a relationship . . . I've wanted to end the relationship a number of times, but then again, I say to myself, take some time, you're overreacting, and say maybe he is doing this because he's dealing with the whole bit and you have to look at it from that respect.

Going Public

This category is defined as managing social relationships and choosing social identification based on information about oneself that is both private and very important. Stages and strategies include (a) Living with secrecy, (b) Asserting oneself, and (c) Balancing risks and benefits. The private and important information focused on the caregiver's involvement with the PWA, and, consequently, his or her association with AIDS. The intent of living with secrecy about one's caregiver status was to protect oneself and the PWA from negative, judgements, rejection, ridicule, and discriminatory acts. Because these consequences could be devastating, caregivers had a vested interest in anticipating others' responses and in planning accordingly.

The uncertainty of *Going Public* involved the inability to predict others' reactions to the knowledge that the caregiver was taking care of a person with AIDS. One mother felt apprehensive about responding to commonplace inquiries from friends and acquaintances.

I really do have a child who is involved in homosexuality, perhaps, and that is not socially acceptable yet. How do I deal with this? . . . My daughter brought this out just last week, and I haven't resolved this issue yet. What am I going to do when I meet a former neighbor or somebody in a grocery store who asks, "How are the kids?"

Because of their inability to predict the reactions of others, caregivers often orchestrated disclosure by carefully choosing who to tell, by making concrete plans for disclosure, and by staging the type and among of information given. One woman spent a considerable amount of time with her friend developing a plan about how together they would inform his family:

His mother had a lot of problems with homosexuality and with his having AIDS. The day before we started telling his family we had structured a whole process of how he would inform his family, who he would tell first. [We would] sort of gain acceptance on the most promising ground and move through a process. And we had this in place, a plan . . .

Containing the Spread of HIV

This subcategory is defined as the fear surrounding the spread of HIV infection and the strategies used to prevent transmission to self and others. Stages and strategies include (a) Confronting fear and personal vulnerability and (b) Doing things differently. Uncertainty about transmission was particularly troubling in the beginning of caregiving. One priest caring for a close friend in a congregate living setting described the initial questions of the group about *Containing the Spread* in response to the PWA's move into the house:

> What do we do with this kind of thing? What does it mean that he's in the public areas of our house? All the fears of AIDS. What does a person with AIDS have to watch out for in terms of hygiene and all those kinds of things? We had a meeting in which everyone [living in the house] sat down and talked to each other about it.

Furthermore, some caregivers lacked confidence in the efficacy of preventive measures and were not always reassured by scientific information alone. One wife caring for her husband expressed her mistrust of "safer sex," and had great difficulty resuming their sexual relationship:

> I know that when I tried to have sex with him I was very fearful. Even though there was protection and everybody told me I was 98% safe, I had fear mixed with a lack of trust, and the whole situation was a great conflict for me.

One lesbian who was caring for her former lover emphasized the particular uncertainty associated with female-to-female transmission:

> I used to always wear gloves during sex and now I don't wear them sometimes. And the rubber dams, just forget it. I go on an intuitive basis pretty much. I really make sure I don't have any cuts on me. I'm a total guinea pig. Nobody knows how women are going to transfer it.

For many partners and spouses, an essential component of confronting fear and vulnerability was facing their own HIV status. Many worried about their own HIV exposure, and uncertainty resurfaced each time they sought periodic AIDS testing. One gay partner described the conflict associated with regular HIV testing:

> It was funny because I got the results of my latest HIV test, and the next day I flew out of Seattle [on business]. And I'm thinking, God, what if this is positive? But it wasn't, thank God . . . And then, once I got the results of the first test back you feel like, I'll live forever. But that doesn't mean a year down the road you won't be. "Oh, no, I thought I was going to escape . . ."

❖ DISCUSSION

Chick and Meleis (1986) identified illness, recovery, and loss (all of which are integral to the AIDS family caregiving phenomenon) as precipitators of transitions. According to Murphy (1990, p. 1), "A transitions perspective is valuable because, to the extent that transitions are anticipatory, preparation for role change and prevention of negative effects can be instituted." Although most authors equate transitions with change, work by Golan (1981) supports the interrelationship between transitions and uncertainty found in this study; she defined transitions as "a period of moving from one state of certainty to another, with an interval of uncertainty and change in between" (p. 12).

Uncertainty has been studied primarily in relation to experiences with chronic or life-threatening illnesses (Mishel, 1988; Mishel & Braden, 1987; Mishel & Braden, 1988; Cohen, 1989), and more recently pregnancy (Sorenson, 1990), breast cancer (Hilton, 1988), and AIDS (Gordon & Shontz, 1990; Weitz, 1989). In a hermeneutical inquiry that examined living with the AIDS virus, Gordon and Shontz (1990) identified uncertainty as a major theme which was closely woven into the other themes of feeling infected and infectious, facing death and dying, secrecy, and ambivalence. Weitz (1989) found that uncertainty in the lives of PWAs focused on the acquisition of AIDS, the meaning of symptoms, short-term functioning, living with dignity, and the prognosis of AIDS. Given the uncertainty experienced by PWAs, it is not surprising that similar concerns regarding uncertainty were prevalent among family members in this study.

While uncertainty has been noted in other caregiving situations, such as cancer, it is a relatively unexplored theme in the family caregiving literature. Research about caregiver uncertainty suggests (a) an association between the uncertainty and caregiver health (Stetz, 1989), (b) uncertainty related to the course of therapy and outcomes resulted in significant caregiver needs (Blank, Clark, Longman, & Atwood, 1989), (c) uncertainty associated with managing the illness and monitoring symptoms was a significant source of stress for parents of chronically ill children (Cohen, 1989), and (d) the early stages of caregiving for the cognitively impaired elderly were marked with uncertainty and unpredictability (Wilson, 1989). Much of the uncertainty in the family caregiving literature was associated with the illness itself, whereas data in the present study revealed that uncertainty in AIDS caregiving also pertained to loss and dying, interpersonal relationships, contagion, and the presentation of self. Furthermore, uncertainty was an important concern for caregivers, similar to the uncertainty reported by family members of cancer patients (Chekryn, 1985; Germino, 1984).

The results advance understanding of AIDS caregiving uncertainty by integrating a theoretical perspective on transitions, by delineating cultural and social contextual features, and by specifying content areas (that is, according to the five caregiving subcategories). Therefore, the findings highlight directions for developing clinical therapeutics in the areas of AIDS family caregiving and uncertainty. Anticipatory guidance could be an important strategy to help caregivers cope with uncertainty because they can identify it, expect it, accept it, and define which of the uncertain circumstances are appropriate and desirable to change. Anticipating caregiving as a transitional period marked by major changes and a new perspective on what is important in life may help reduce the strain associated with the demands of caregiving. In considering clinical therapeutics for AIDS family caregivers, significant gaps remain in understanding the content and timing of the most appropriate interventions. Longitudinal research designs are best suited to address these gaps because of the transitional nature of caregiving as it changes over time. Longitudinal data about

AIDS family caregiving are essential to refine the content and timing of interventions to maximize therapeutic value, and to enhance cost-effectiveness.

References

Baumgarten, M. (1989). The health of a person giving care to the demented elderly: A critical review of literature. *Journal of Clinical Epidemiology, 42,* 1137–1148.

Blank, J. J., Clark, L., Longman, A. J., & Atwood, J. R. (1989). Perceived home care needs of cancer patients and their caregivers. *Cancer Nursing, 12*(2), 78–84.

Blumer, H. (1969). *Symbolic interactionism: Perspective and method.* Englewood Cliffs, NJ: Prentice Hall.

Bosers, B. (1987). Intergenerational caregiving: Adult caregivers and their aging parents. *Advances in Nursing Science, 9*(2), 20–31.

Chekryn, J. (1984). Cancer recurrence: Personal meaning, communication and marital adjustment. *Cancer Nursing, 7,* 491–498.

Chenoweth, B., & Spencer, B. (1986). Dementia: The experience of family caregivers. *The Gerontologist, 26,* 267–272.

Chick, N., & Meleis, A. I. (1986). Transitions: A nursing concern. In P. L. Chinn (Ed.), *Nursing research methodology* (pp. 237–257). Rockville, MD: Aspen.

Cohen, M. H. (1989). The sources and management of uncertainty in life-threatening chronic illness [Abstract]. *Communicating Nursing Research, 22,* 155.

DSHS & Seattle-King County Health Department. (1991). *Washington ST/Seattle-King County HIV/AIDS Epidemiology Report,* 1st quarter, p. 1.

Edwards, B. (1988). Stories from the front: How to cope when your lover has ARC or AIDS. In T. Eidson (Ed.), *The AIDS caregiver's handbook* (pp. 206–216). New York: St. Martin's Press.

Ekberg, J., Griffith, N., & Foxall, M. J. (1986). Spouse burnout syndrome. *Journal of Advanced Nursing, 1,* 161–165.

Germino, B. B. (1984). *Family members' concerns after cancer diagnosis.* Unpublished doctoral dissertation, University of Washington, Seattle.

Glaser, B., & Strauss, A. (1967). *The discovery of grounded theory: Strategies for qualitative research.* Chicago: Aldine.

Golan, N. (1981). *Passing through transitions.* New York: Free Press.

Gordon, J., & Shontz, F. (1990). Living with the AIDS virus: A representative case. *Journal of Counseling and Development, 68,* 287–292.

Haque, R. (1989). A family's experience with AIDS. In J. H. Flaskerud (Ed.), *AIDS/HIV Infection: A reference guide for nursing professionals* (pp. 230–240). Philadelphia: W. B. Saunders.

Hepburn, K. (1990). Informal caregivers: Front-line workers in the chronic care of AIDS patients. In *Community based care for persons with AIDS: Developing a research agenda* (pp. 37–42), (DHHS Publication No. (PHS) 90-3456). Washington, DC: U.S. Government Printing Office.

Hilton, B. A. (1988). The phenomenon of uncertainty in women with breast cancer. *Issues in Mental Health Nursing, 9,* 217–238.

Lincoln, Y. S., & Guba, E. G. (1985). *Naturalistic inquiry.* Beverly Hills, CA: Sage.

Livingston, M. (1985). Families who care. *British Medical Journal, 291,* 919–920.

Miller, B., & Montgomery, A. (1990). Family caregivers and limitations in social activities. *Research on Aging, 12,* 72–93.

Mishel, M. (1990). Reconceptualization of the Uncertainty in Illness theory. *IMAGE: Journal of Nursing Scholarship, 22,* 256–262.

Mishel, M. (1988). Uncertainty in illness. *Image, 20,* 225–232.

Mishel, M., & Braden, C. (1987). Uncertainty: A mediator between support and adjustment. *Western Journal of Nursing Research, 9,* 43–57.

Mishel, M., & Braden, M. (1988). Finding meaning: Antecedents of uncertainty in illness. *Nursing Research, 37,* 98–103.

Moffatt, B. C. (1986). *When someone you love has AIDS.* New York: NAL Penguin.

Monette, P. (1988). *Borrowed time.* New York: Avon Books.

Montgomery, R., Gonyea, J., & Hooyman, N. (1985). Caregiving and the experience of subjective and objective burden. *Family Relations, 34,* 19–26.

Murphy, S. A. (1990). Human responses to transitions: A holistic nursing perspective. *Holistic Nursing Practice, 4*(3), 1–7.

Ostrow, D., & Gayle, T. (1986). Psychosocial and ethical issues of AIDS health care programs. *Quarterly Review Bulletin, 12,* 284–294.

Parkes, C. M. (1971). Psycho-social transitions: A field for study. *Social Science & Medicine, 5,* 101–115.

Rabins, P. V., Mace, N. L., & Lucas, M. J. (1982). The impact of dementia on the family. *Journal of the American Medical Association, 248,* 333–335.

Rabins, P. V., Fitting, M. D., Eastham, J., & Fetting, J. (1990). The emotional impact of caring for the chronically ill. *Psychosomatics, 31,* 331–336.

Raveis, V., & Siegel, K. (1990). Impact of caregiving on informal or familial caregivers. In *Community-based care of persons with AIDS: Developing a research agenda* (pp. 17–28). (DHHS Publication Number (PHS) 90-3456). Washington, DC: U.S. Printing Office.

Sandelowski, M. (1986). The problem of rigor in qualitative research. *Advances in Nursing Science, 8*(3), 27–37.

Schoen, K. (1986). Psychosocial aspects of hospice care for AIDS patients. *The American Journal of Hospice Care, 3*(2), 32–34.

Shilts, R. (1987). *And the band played on: Politics, people, and the AIDS epidemic.* New York: St. Martin's Press.

Snyder, B., & Keefe, K. (1985). The unmet needs of family caregivers for frail and disabled adults. *Social Work in Health Care, 10*(3), 1–14.

Sorenson, D. (1990). Uncertainty in pregnancy. NAACOG's *Clinical Issues in Perinatal and Women's Health Nursing, 1,* 289–296.

Stetz, K. (1989). The relationship among background characteristics, purpose in life, and caregiving demands on perceived health of spouse caregivers. *Scholarly Inquiry for Nursing Practice, 3,* 133–159.

Strauss, A. L. (1987). *Qualitative analysis for social scientists.* Cambridge: Cambridge University Press.

Thomas, R. (1987). Family adaptation to a child with a chronic condition. In M. H. Rose & R. B. Thomas (Eds.), *Children with chronic conditions* (pp. 29–54). New York: Harcourt Brace Jovanovich.

Weitz, R. (1989). Uncertainty and the lives of persons with AIDS. *Journal of Health and Social Behavior, 30,* 270–281.

Wilson, H. S. (1989). Family caregiving for a relative with Alzheimer's dementia: Coping with negative choices. *Nursing Research, 38,* 94–98.

Wolcott, D. L., Fawzy, F. I., & Landsverk, J., & McCombs, M. (1986). AIDS patients' needs of psychosocial services and their use of community service organizations. *Journal of Psychosocial Oncology, 4,* 135–146.

Zarit, S. H., Todd, P. A., & Zarit, J. M. (1986). Subjective burden of husbands and wives as caregivers. A longitudinal study. *The Gerontologist, 26,* 260–266.